BE KIND,

BE CALM,

BE SAFE

ALSO BY DR. BONNIE HENRY

*Soap and Water and
Common Sense*

Be Kind, Be Calm, Be Safe

Four Weeks That Shaped a Pandemic

**Dr. Bonnie Henry &
Lynn Henry**

ALLEN
LANE

ALLEN LANE
an imprint of Penguin Canada,
a division of Penguin Random House Canada Limited

Canada • USA • UK • Ireland • Australia • New Zealand •
India • South Africa • China

First published 2021

www.penguinrandomhouse.ca

LIBRARY AND ARCHIVES CANADA CATALOGUING IN PUBLICATION

Title: Be kind, be calm, be safe : four weeks that shaped a pandemic /
Bonnie Henry, Lynn Henry.
Names: Henry, Bonnie, Dr., author. | Henry, Lynn, author.
Identifiers: Canadiana (print) 20200310267 | Canadiana (ebook) 20200310984 |
ISBN 9780735241855 (hardcover) | ISBN 9780735241862 (EPUB)
Subjects: LCSH: Henry, Bonnie, Dr. | LCSH: Henry, Lynn. | LCSH: British
Columbia. Office of the Provincial Health Officer—Officials and employees—
Biography. | LCSH: Health officers—British Columbia—Biography. | LCSH:
Sisters—British Columbia—Biography. | LCSH: COVID-19 (Disease)—British
Columbia. | LCSH: Epidemics—British Columbia—History—21st century. |
LCGFT: Autobiographies.
Classification: LCC RA424.5.H46 A3 2021 | DDC 362.1092—dc23

Cover and book design by Jennifer Griffiths
Cover image © Jackie Dives

Printed and bound in Canada

10 9 8 7 6 5 4 3 2

 Penguin
Random
House

To our elders and caregivers.
And for our sisters.

CONTENTS

PROLOGUE

*"I Ask This Global Community
to Pause"*

IN LYNN HENRY'S WORDS

Sometimes you don't see the warning until it's too late. Sometimes you hear the warning but fail to heed its message. And sometimes you see, hear, *and* understand— but the symphonic roar of the world drowns out your solo note of alarm. A single tragedy unites us all in the end, though: our many small, casual, disbelieving, distracted, unsure, risk-calculated, understandable, self-serving, self-sacrificing, protective, recalcitrant, completely unaware, and very particular failures to see, hear, and communicate reveal their true meaning only on the other side of the impassable divide between "then" and "now."

This story begins with the end of "then."

On New Year's Eve, as 2019 was silently, invisibly mutating into 2020, my sister Bonnie and I were, unusually, together. Normally I would have flown to Prince Edward Island from Toronto, where I live, to spend the holidays with my parents there. And Bonnie habitually spent the same period in her beloved home of British Columbia, where two years earlier she had been appointed the province's "top doctor," or medical officer of health—the first woman to hold that position. The last time we'd spent New Year's in each other's company had been more than twenty years before, when Bonnie was in San Diego, finishing a degree in public health and working as a family doctor at an inner-city medical clinic. I had joined her from Canada that long-ago December, and I remember visiting the clinic one afternoon and Bonnie calmly pointing out the pockmarks of bullet holes in a waiting-room wall. She explained that the building housing the clinic happened to sit at an intersection between the streets of rival gangs. Occasionally there would be drive-by shootings, and staff and patients would duck for cover, make sure there were no casualties outside or in, and carry on.

As 2019 shape-shifted into 2020, however, Bonnie and I were seemingly as far away from that earlier time and space as you could get, sitting quietly on a balcony under a slim crescent moon, overlooking a cliff that sloped down to the Caribbean Sea. Our uncle had for decades owned a suite in the beautiful old hotel where we were staying, and out of the blue he had offered us the space for ten days during this quietest time of year; he, like most of the regulars, would arrive for a much longer stretch in late January, escaping the wintry Prairies. Bonnie had been exhausted in drizzly Victoria, I was bone-weary in grey Toronto, and we'd both perked up equally at this surprise invitation. Now, six days in, we sat outside in the soft dark as Bonnie told me tales of her time on this very island years earlier—while still in medical school, she and a windsurf-loving colleague had spent a semester learning and practising emergency medicine at a hospital in the nearby capital city, travelling the coast in search of waves on their days off.

Just before midnight, we sipped a celebratory whisky in companionable silence. I listened to the sea breaking against the cliff-foot, thinking how the sound was so very strange in this moment, yet as familiar to me as breath, just as my sister's presence on this particular day was so strange and familiar all at once, our lives like two strands in a helix mysteriously crossing at key points; and I was reminded of our parents on another fragile island, no doubt frozen and blustery just then, in the North Atlantic. I thought, too, of the prime minister of this place whose waves were right now a calm, regular rhythm in my ears, the extraordinary Mia Mottley, and her unsettling, searing words a year before to the UN about the plight of small island nations in our time of climate change. "In good conscience, I cannot give the speech that I prepared," she had told the world then, as she arranged to cut her trip short and rush home to deal with devastating storms and severe flooding. "We, as a small state, are used to being treated as if we didn't exist . . . [But] what happened in the last twenty-four hours is not a science fiction movie. We must have caring and empathy . . . It is not about governments anymore," she said. "It is about people. I ask this global community to pause. Time is running out."

"I'm worried about what will happen next year," Bonnie said suddenly into the night sky, as if spying the trail of my thoughts. "The health minister and I haven't talked directly for a while. That's my responsibility, too, of course. But we need to align our ideas on how to communicate about the overdose crisis."

On cue, a loud alarm started up, its siren interrupting her words. We both stood and leaned over the balcony, peering at the pool belonging to the ground-floor suite below. Its water rippled in the light breeze, but otherwise pool and suite appeared undisturbed and empty, as they had been all week. Still the siren continued, harsh and insistent. "Well, something's set it off," Bonnie said. "Maybe an animal tripped it. I'll call the front desk and ask if security might check it out and hopefully make it stop."

As I looked past the glow of underwater lights around the edge of the pool into the darker waving shadows of the tall grasses leading to the edge of the cliff, another, perhaps ridiculous, possibility occurred to me. "I think it might be frogs," I ventured. "Not an alarm at all."

Bonnie shook her head. "No, definitely not. I'm calling the night desk."

I admire Bonnie's characteristic certainty, a quality she has possessed since childhood, because I know it's informed by a clear-eyed understanding of the facts and a measured consideration of the probabilities. I weighed this against my own way of seeing and mulling multiple competing possibilities at once. Usually, in our relationship, mine was the losing proposition. "Humour me?" I said after a pause, and perhaps it was the smoky whisky or the beckoning warmth of the air or the worry that I would set off stubbornly on my own, but Bonnie sighed and did.

Soon we were scrambling through thorny hedges and high grass. We reached a clearing, and I stooped to find a rock, the siren now on a dreadful, ever-louder repeating loop. With little hope, I flung the rock in the direction of the cliff and heard a dull *thunk*. Then: magnificent silence. Bonnie and I each held an inhalation for a long moment—and the silence held, too. In the final seconds of the old year, we laughed and laughed, relieved and a little embarrassed as we made our way back, only the sound of the sea exhaling behind us.

But somewhere, I know now, there really was an alarm ringing. I just couldn't hear its unusual frequency, whereas my sister—her senses heightened by a nimbus of PTSD from her experience twenty years earlier fighting SARS; by her current pitch of constant anxiety, honed over the past year's desperate, and frankly losing, fight to control the overdose crisis raging in her province; and by her never-sleeping internal weather system that was already gathering and synthesizing still-cloudy signs and signals coming out of the World Health Organization—could.

In less than a month, back in Canada, she and her province's health minister, now in almost daily contact, would hold their first joint press conference about a stealthy new virus spreading breath by breath throughout the world.

IN DR. BONNIE HENRY'S WORDS

M ost of us go through our days blissfully unaware of the constant small cues the world sends out about potential hazards that may invade our lives: heat alerts that could translate into wildfires raging out of control; weather advisories that may morph into hurricanes and storm surges; recall notifications of salmonella-laced spinach whose consumption might lead to hundreds being sickened. For those of us on the frontlines of public health, though, these are the modern tickertapes that flow through our days. Whether they're alerts on the global PROMED listserv that tell of unusual cases and outbreaks of illness in all corners of the globe or random online articles that mention a doctor in China raising an alarm, we follow these signs carefully—and perhaps, for some of us, with something akin to religious fanaticism. As we watch the world move en masse and people go about their daily business, these signs pop up in our consciousness as warnings. But which ones are signals of something bigger, more ominous?

That is the challenge and the work of public health experts across the globe. We watch the signs in our local communities;

in our provinces, states, or regions; in our countries; and collectively around the world through the World Health Organization. We're a minuscule part of the health system in countries everywhere, and mostly behind the scenes, but we're also essential, preventing illness and injury, protecting and promoting health in all its forms. And every now and then we emerge from the shadows to play a critical role, leading the response to threats that can range from influenza to Ebola, to food-borne illness, to lead in drinking water, to the effects of climate change and radiation. In these moments, public health teams globally become the front lines.

You may not realize it, but when you develop such symptoms as the characteristic cough and fever of influenza and seek care from your local doctor, at that moment you may enter an international network set up to monitor the spread of key infections and detect new pathogens, whether it's a novel strain of influenza or something completely different. Our surveillance systems include laboratories around the world that submit data to the WHO on the genomic makeup of influenza viruses circulating in their local areas, the monitoring of emergency department visits for "influenza-like illness" (ILI), and the tracking of clusters and outbreaks of ILI in settings like long-term care homes, hospitals, and schools. We also have systems that detect whether people with severe pneumonias or other serious illnesses are being admitted to hospitals or to intensive care units—what we call SARI surveillance, for "severe acute respiratory illness." We trace the patterns and monitor the cases in an ongoing, systematic way so that when something new and different shows up, we can detect it.

In Canada, with our universal health coverage, we're also able to track important markers like physician visits for ILI. All these measures alert us to when the annual influenza season is starting and help us monitor its severity and geographic spread as it progresses through the winter. On a weekly basis, public health experts like me receive these data in the form of reports that compare what we're seeing this week to averages from the last ten or more years. This helps us put the data in perspective and determine whether there's something unusual that we need to investigate. We look at three basic characteristics—person, place, and time—to determine if there's anything out of the ordinary. This means we assess whether there's a cluster of people—for example, people of the same age or in the same city within a short period of time—who are affected, which could be a signal that we need to investigate. Many times, these investigations lead nowhere and the cluster is just chance, but sometimes those signals do lead to something more worrisome.

Seasonal influenza is one of the illnesses we track relentlessly. The measures we take to understand its spread through populations and across geographic regions, to prevent its transmission, and to investigate and control its outbreaks are also a yearly test of our ability to track the global spread of a new illness—in other words, to detect and respond to a pandemic. Our annual influenza immunization campaigns test our ability to vaccinate large numbers of people in all communities in a short period of time. They also help people *understand* the vaccine and the importance of infection prevention and control measures, from hand washing to mask wearing in hospitals and long-term care facilities to staying home when you're sick. Many of the simple things we do to fight the flu every year work just as well to prevent transmission of all respiratory viruses to our families, friends, and communities.

In short, public health surveillance is much more than just counting illnesses. It is the systematic, ongoing collection of these data, followed by analysis to understand what story the data tells, and finally communication of that information to those who make decisions and take action. It is the system that underpins the work public health teams do every day in detecting threats to health in our communities and taking action to contain and prevent further illness.

And it's not just influenza we track; many illnesses fall under our surveillance. By law, these "reportable communicable diseases," or RCDs, must be reported to public health by the clinician or lab that has made the diagnosis. Most of these diseases belong to our long history of plagues and pestilences that have affected human populations for centuries: scourges like measles, polio, and tuberculosis, as well as the many illnesses we have immunization programs to prevent, including bacterial meningitis and hepatitis B. Some of these diseases are new—mosquito-borne illnesses like Zika and West Nile virus infection, and the devastating viral hemorrhagic fevers caused by Ebola virus. Some are transmitted through food and water, like salmonella and Cyclospora, or through sexual contact, like HIV or syphilis. In all, there are about sixty RCDs that are required by law to be reported to public health in provinces and territories in Canada. Very similar lists exist in countries across the globe. The monitoring of these key illnesses is a silent safety net spread out around the world so that if something alarming is happening, we can detect it, trace it, and take action against it.

What all RCDs have in common are the public health interventions we can take to stop or control transmission, or prevent people in close contact with a case from getting sick themselves. Public health experts—mainly physicians known as medical officers of health, as well as public health nurses and inspectors—collect this information and contact the affected individuals to make sure they're getting the support they need for the illness and are taking actions necessary to prevent its transmission to others. This could mean providing immunization or an antibiotic to someone who's been exposed—to measles, meningitis, or hepatitis B, for example—so that they can develop antibodies or receive the medication to protect them from getting sick. It's a highly effective procedure for many vaccine-preventable illnesses, but timing is critical: generally, post-exposure immunization or prophylaxis needs to happen within days of an exposure. For this reason, quick reporting is key to effective prevention of outbreaks in these cases. Time truly is of the essence.

For other illnesses like salmonella, reporting of cases leads to public health investigations to determine whether, for example, a common food source is contaminated. Public health detective work has identified many different food-borne outbreaks in everything from onions and almonds to milk and hamburgers. Identification of contaminated foods can in turn lead to recalls and to improved farming conditions or other actions that prevent future outbreaks. Again, timing is important: we need to make sure that the culprit is taken out of circulation before more people get sick.

While most diseases are reportable to public health at a local level, some are also reported at a national level, and still others need to be understood on a global scale. These latter are reported to the WHO by all countries in the World Health Association according to what are known as the International Health Regulations, or IHR. For many decades the IHR required the reporting of only three specific illnesses: smallpox, yellow fever, and cholera. Smallpox, in a global public health triumph, was eradicated worldwide in the late 1970s, and both yellow fever and cholera are rare, particularly in most Western nations. But then, in the early 2000s, something changed.

IN 2003 A NEW WARNING sign appeared—and it became clear that the world needed to keep its sights fixed on more than just three pathogens.

That year, reports of a severe, atypical pneumonia from clinicians in Guangzhou, China, sent ripples of worry across the globe. "Atypical pneumonia" is medical code for a serious respiratory infection, cause unknown. People were getting sick with a lung infection that put them in hospital, and some were dying. No one could determine the cause. But then the official word came from Beijing: it was *Chlamydia pneumoniae*. There had been 340 cases and five deaths. It was all under control. Nothing to see here.

Chlamydia is indeed a bacterium that can cause a type of pneumonia, but this explanation seemed highly unlikely to the people who study these things. Around that time we'd been hearing reports of a new strain of influenza also causing illness in China, known as influenza A H5N1. Many of us thought the mystery illness was much more likely to be a new, potentially dangerous influenza virus—and we started to prepare.

Rumours continued to surface despite repeated denials from the Beijing government. This was especially true in Hong Kong, a city uniquely positioned to see what was happening in China— and uniquely at risk. Soon enough, a travelling physician unwittingly brought the new illness from his hospital in Guangzhou to Hong Kong. He became ill in a hotel there, and guests who had contact with him in the elevator, in the breakfast room, and in the hallways picked it up, too. Within days, the disease began its destructive journey to countries around the world, from Singapore to Vietnam to Taiwan to Toronto, where I was working as a medical officer of health. When our first cases were detected in Toronto, we still didn't know what was causing this new and severe illness. It still didn't have a name, a test, or a treatment. Nor did we know exactly how it was spread, or even whether its cause was a virus at all.

That atypical pneumonia, we soon learned, was indeed caused by a coronavirus—one that came to be known around the world as SARS. By the end of 2003 it had infected 8098 people globally and killed 744, but by then we'd pushed the virus back into nature: a tremendous feat with tremendous cost. I witnessed then, unforgettably, how SARS brought out the worst and best in human nature, allowing prejudices and biases to be widely exposed in ways many ordinary citizens hadn't seen before while also allowing for moments of great sacrifice, compassion, and grace.

SARS was also a warning.

The many global inquiries that later dissected the outbreak, after the virus had been controlled, all pointed to China's failure to notify the world of what was happening within its borders as being particularly egregious. That failure had deprived the global community of precious time in which we could have both assisted and prepared. China committed to doing better. And it was evident to all that the International Health Regulations, as they currently existed, needed to be revised and expanded so that the obligations of all countries to global awareness would be made clear. The revamped IHR came out in 2005, and this binding instrument of international law came into force on June 15, 2007.

It might not seem rational to hide an outbreak of an infectious disease, but in fact there are, tragically, very justified fears that if a nation reports something that has the potential to spread, trade and travel to and from that country could be severely affected—which could, of course, lead to unnecessary hardship and economic losses. We'd seen this before. When an outbreak of bubonic and pneumonic plague hit parts of India in 1994, there was global panic. It started in late August when health officials in Surat, in Gujarat state, reported large numbers of deaths of local rats. Soon after, a human case of plague was reported to the local health officer, along with reports of as many as fifty seriously ill people being admitted to hospital in the city. Within days, as news spread, more than 300,000 people fled Surat, afraid of the disease but equally afraid of being quarantined in the "plague city." By the time the outbreak was over, 693 cases and fifty-six deaths had been reported from five Indian states and the city of Delhi. No cases had been exported outside of India. Around the world, however, fear of the illness's potential spread led to flight cancellations and restrictions on the movement of goods. All of this had severe economic and health impacts on people across India that lasted for years.

And in 1997, an outbreak of a novel influenza strain, Avian Influenza H5N1, in the wet markets of Hong Kong led to the culling of more than 1.5 million chickens and severely curtailed travel and the movement of goods to and from the island nation. In the end the virus was contained, with infection confirmed in only eighteen people and, unfortunately, six deaths. It was, however, a wake-up call to the world about the very real possibility of a coming influenza pandemic.

After SARS, China responded swiftly and positively to the new IHR by dramatically increasing research into coronaviruses and committing to more timely responses and openness with the WHO. Indeed, in the years since SARS, much of the world's knowledge of coronaviruses has been developed in China—where several large research teams investigate everything from the viruses' natural hosts (likely bats) to the spillover into animal and human populations to their genetic variances. In particular, the Chinese research teams developed banks of viral genomic sequences associated with different animal species, focusing on those animals linked to the transmission to humans—especially the illegally traded wild animals so common in many Chinese wet markets. This new research was added to an existing strong investigative program that had been studying influenza viruses for years. And there were good indications of the country's increased openness, with several novel influenza variants being promptly reported to the WHO by Chinese authorities and then well managed.

EVEN BEFORE SARS, COUNTRIES around the world had been preparing for a pandemic for years—and it was influenza that was generally considered to be the most likely cause. Influenza is a virus that has afflicted human populations for centuries. Circling the globe annually, it preys on the young and the elderly, leading to thousands of deaths worldwide every year. Because the influenza virus has only one strand of nuclear material (RNA) making up its eight small genes, it can change rapidly and take on new bits of genetic material from the cells it infects. The influenza virus changes just enough that the human immune system no longer recognizes it, meaning a new vaccine must be developed to combat the new form of the virus each year. But the influenza virus can also change dramatically at short notice by exchanging a gene or a large piece of several genes with other influenza viruses—and this can lead to major pandemics. A *pandemic* is a disease that circles the world, affecting people in many countries in a short period of time; this is in contrast to an *epidemic* or an *outbreak*, the terms we use for diseases that cause illness in smaller areas at a time. Our seasonal epidemics of influenza affect regions of the globe in a predictable pattern in the winter months of each hemisphere: typically, October to March in the northern hemisphere and June to September in the southern hemisphere. The WHO estimates that 5 to 15 percent of the world's population is affected by influenza every year, with three to five million severe cases requiring medical attention and hospitalization, and 250,000 to 500,000 cases resulting in death.

In the past century and a half, a major global outbreak, or pandemic, of influenza has occurred about every forty years and affected millions. The Spanish Flu of 1918–1919, however, still stands out as the most devastating influenza pandemic in world history. Its occurrence at the tail end of the First World War meant that it spread rapidly among returning troops and through victory celebrations in populations still reeling from years of war and suffering. Estimates vary, but even conservative ones suggest that the Spanish influenza pandemic killed forty million people around the world. It was the spectre of a reoccurrence of such devastation that focused our attention on influenza and pandemic preparedness.

After SARS, the WHO raised the alarm once again: we needed to prepare for future pandemics, and that included developing plans that would support all the countries of the world. Canada, fresh from its searing experience with SARS, was a leader in this initiative and one of the first nations to publish a nationwide influenza pandemic plan that covered such issues as scaling up laboratory testing, determining the most at-risk populations, and arranging for mass casualties and mass vaccinations.

By then we had another tool in fighting influenza: antiviral medications that can lessen the impact of the virus as well as decrease the time one is infectious—and so we put plans in place for stockpiling these, too. Influenza really is the quintessential virus for pandemic planners, because to prepare for an influenza pandemic you have to consider everything from the overall structure of the response, to lab testing, surveillance, and epidemiology, to the delivery of vaccines and treatments. Thinking about an influenza pandemic also forced us to address such fraught issues as protocols for international travel; the closing of borders, businesses, and schools; impacts on the global economy and trade; and the critical societal issues of equity of access to essential services and medications. In the global public health world, we were convinced that preparing for the spread of influenza would stand us in good stead no matter what microbe caused the next pandemic.

As internet and social media sites flourished across China after the 2003 SARS outbreak, scientists from around the world who were interested in respiratory viruses, primarily influenza, were able to connect with each other in a whole new virtual way, exchanging information on what was happening in their communities and what they were seeing in their labs and hospitals. Scientists, public health experts, epidemiologists, and clinicians in this informal network communicated on a regular basis about what was happening in the "flu world," whether it was news of a variant detected in agricultural fairs in the United States or novel strains picked up in markets in Hong Kong.

In 2009, the first signals of a new influenza virus sickening people in Mexico came out of this network and raised the alarm. This same virus was soon detected in the U.S. and Canada, with outbreaks detected in rapid succession in California, a boarding school in Nova Scotia, and a remote northern community in British Columbia. The event we'd spent years preparing for had come to pass: an influenza pandemic. Eventually labelled "Influenza A pandemic HINI-2009," the outbreak spread around the globe within weeks, stretching affected countries' ability to respond. But the lessons from SARS were still relatively fresh, and this new virus was influenza, which we'd studied thoroughly—so the response was swift, a test was available in days, the epidemiology was worked out, and a vaccine was developed in months.

When the influenza A HINI pandemic began in Mexico, the IHR was the instrument used to coordinate actions and notifications internationally. And for the most part, this new protocol worked. The WHO managed the response at the global level and convened expert groups to provide guidance for countries on surveillance, use of personal protective equipment, and use of antivirals and vaccines.

The 2009 pandemic challenged many of our assumptions and forced us to be nimble in ways that hadn't always been anticipated, but by and large the planning held true. There was, of course, the initial chaos and scramble to understand the particularities of a new deadly infection: Who would be most at risk, how would we get treatment to those who needed it, would we have enough ventilators, and how would decisions be made about the allocation of scarce resources? Who would make them? And how long would a vaccine take, would it be safe, would it be effective? How many waves would there be? What would be the impact on low- and middle-income countries compared to wealthier ones? The pandemic also exposed inequities globally and within countries—who was affected most by the measures put in place to control the virus, who had access to vaccines or even healthcare, and the effects of the virus on Indigenous populations, with their history of decimation in pandemics past.

In the end, though, this influenza behaved much like the influenzas we knew and had studied. Young people were most widely affected, but the illness was mostly mild to moderate in children and more severe in adults. In a surprise twist, many older people, especially those over eighty (those most at risk every year with seasonal influenza epidemics), were less at risk of infection, likely because they'd gained immunity from having been exposed to a similar influenza virus in their youth. Ultimately, pandemic HINI-2009 likely infected around 700 million people around the world and, sadly, caused an estimated 280,000 deaths—numbers similar to those of a bad seasonal influenza epidemic. The vaccine was developed rapidly, and by the fall of 2009, mass immunization around the world had led to dramatic decreases in infections and stopped the pandemic in its tracks. The vaccine turned out to be highly effective and safe. By the time the 2010 Winter Olympic Games began in Vancouver in February, HINI influenza was gone completely and the Games were a virus-free celebration. Despite the disruptions, sickness, distressing deaths, and uncertainty—and the recriminations and public inquiries that followed—the world had come through pandemic HINI-2009 relatively unscathed.

The WHO had played a key role in this but nonetheless came under intense scrutiny and criticism during and after the 2009 pandemic. In subsequent years, budgets were cut and the focus of WHO programs moved on to address chronic disease and other key millennium development goals. Pandemic preparedness and the emergency response program, including the Global Outbreak Alert and Response Network (known by the ungainly acronym GOARN) teams, languished. There were even claims that we on the front lines of public health had overreacted, that the WHO had been too influenced by vaccine manufacturers. Some people asserted that scientists thoroughly understood influenza now, that the global risk was exaggerated. And perhaps it's true that we came through with a sense of complacency, that we thought we knew how to deal with influenza, that we were convinced we'd never see anything like the 1918 pandemic again. We knew too much; we had modern systems for testing, treatment, and vaccines. *We've got this*, we said.

AS THE WHO REFOCUSED and nations around the world reviewed their 2009 pandemic response, our next global crisis emerged seemingly out of the blue. This time it came in the form of an Ebola outbreak that, beginning in 2014, wreaked havoc on some of the poorest countries on the planet: Côte d'Ivoire, Guinea, and Liberia. Previous Ebola outbreaks had arisen in more remote areas of what was then called Zaire (now the Democratic Republic of the Congo), Sudan, and Uganda, all in sub-Saharan Africa.

I'd worked on the response to what was up till then the largest outbreak in Uganda, in 2000–2001, and knew well the challenges this fearful virus inflicts on families and communities. It's not just the disease Ebola causes when it attacks the blood vessels of the body, leading to bleeding and sometimes rapid death. There's also a fear and stigma disproportionate to the virus's effects, and it is this that leads to communities being overwhelmed and unable to care for their most vulnerable. The 2014–2016 outbreak in West Africa was the largest and most complex since the Ebola virus was first discovered in 1976, with more cases and more deaths than all others combined. It also spread between countries, starting in Guinea then moving across land borders to Sierra Leone and Liberia. And it caught the WHO's response teams by surprise. Lacking in resources, its response was slow, as was the response globally—leaving the affected countries strained to breaking and marginalized.

Once the world realized the dangers, however, a concerted effort by the global community eventually controlled the virus. Out of this, once again, changes at the WHO followed, this time to shore up its emergency program and bring in the needed expertise to lead a global response. GOARN was revamped and countries recommitted, at least on paper and in the World Health Assembly venues, to preparedness and global solidarity.

We'd dodged another bullet. Despite the devastation and countless deaths, Ebola had not spread around the world, and a pandemic had been averted.

PARADOXICALLY, AMONG THE MOST challenging developments in the immediate aftermath of the 2009 pandemic was a diminution of faith in public health globally, including a rising distrust in vaccines, particularly influenza immunization. Despite (or perhaps because of) the success of the pandemic vaccine, there was a sense that, as I mentioned, the risk of pandemic HINI-2009 had been overblown. In addition, fears had arisen during the pandemic that those who'd been immunized with the previous season's vaccine may have been more likely to become infected with the pandemic strain. While

scientists debated in medical journals the validity of and rationale for such fears, seeds of doubt took root in the larger world.
Anti-vaccine activists exploited the sentiment with propaganda
about vaccine risks and the "compromised" WHO, asserting
that vaccine manufacturers were profiting from the pandemic
and that the vaccine caused more deaths than the virus itself.
This was patently untrue, but the loud bell of concern had
been rung. In the two years following the pandemic, influenza
immunization rates among healthcare workers plummeted
alarmingly—blunting one of the key weapons we possessed for
protecting our most vulnerable people in long-term care homes
and hospitals, and for keeping healthcare workers healthy and
able to work during the annual influenza epidemics.

It was a discouraging development. We in public health
had been working for years to build confidence in influenza
immunization and to stress the importance of the protection
it provides for all. But now a new scientific discourse led some
to doubt the benefits, if not the safety, of seasonal influenza
vaccines. Some scientists felt that these vaccines' protective
benefits had been overstated and their trials biased: that
instead of being 70 to 90 percent effective, their ability to protect a person against influenza more likely stood at 40 to 60
percent, and that this wasn't good enough. These scientists
advocated for more research and effort to go into developing
better vaccines. This important nuance was lost, however. The
message was co-opted by anti-vaccine groups, who claimed
that the vaccines we had were not only ineffective but unsafe.

Meanwhile, we were rapidly learning more and more about
the influenza virus, in particular the way different strains affect
different populations—all of which allowed us to be more effective in our responses. We understood that the influenza A H3N2

virus strain, for example, attacked the elderly most seriously, and that when these viruses predominated we could expect a severe season, with outbreaks and illness and deaths among seniors in both the community and in long-term care. Influenza A H1N1, by contrast, more often hit the young, and when *it* predominated we'd see more children and young adults affected with lots of illness but many fewer deaths. Then there were the influenza B strains that again seemed to cause more illness and spread rapidly among children while causing relatively less disease in older populations.

The other challenge with influenza immunization is the paradox that those most at risk for severe disease or complications from influenza are the same people who don't respond as well to the vaccine. Even healthy seniors, for example, have less response to immunization because our immune system weakens naturally as we age.

In the years following the 2009 pandemic, immunization rates for seasonal influenza fell, precipitously in some places. Most concerningly, rates in healthcare workers fell below levels that would provide the necessary buffer for our most vulnerable in long-term care and hospitals. The relatively mild pandemic and, in some cases, a misinterpretation of the scientific debate had eroded confidence in this important measure—and those who were most vulnerable were put at risk.

Soon this led to a groundswell of initiatives by public health and healthcare organizations to increase immunization rates and protective measures, particularly in healthcare settings. In many places these took the form of "vaccinate or mask" (VOM) policies, whereby during the influenza season healthcare workers were required to be immunized or wear a surgical mask when in patient care areas. The purpose of the mask was to contain a person's secretions in case they'd contracted influenza and were infectious to others in the day or so before symptoms began. This was a compromise. Immunization is by far the better protection—effective not only in the healthcare setting but also in the community, where you're much more likely to contract influenza from your children, family, or friends.

And while the protection a person received from immunization might be as low as 40 percent in some seasons, depending on the virus strain, that was still an important risk reduction individually—and more importantly, it helped curb the spread of the virus in the community, too. If the virus is less likely to encounter susceptible people when someone coughs or sneezes, it can't spread. This is the concept of population or community protection, otherwise known by the slightly less palatable term "herd immunity." With influenza, the more people who are immunized, even with an imperfect vaccine, the more the field of protection increases—and this can prevent outbreaks and infections in those most at risk. But we have no mandatory immunization policies in Canada, and the thought was that making immunization a condition of employment in the healthcare setting was a step too far. The option of wearing a mask instead was a compromise that still put the safety of patients and residents first.

Although many jurisdictions—in the United States in particular, but also around the world—were moving ahead with VOM policies or immunization as a condition of employment in healthcare, it was still controversial. In my province of British Columbia, the implementation of the first province-wide vaccinate-or-mask policy in 2011–2012 was not without its significant challenges. Grievances were filed by most of the healthcare unions on behalf of their members who didn't want to be immunized nor to wear masks. They argued that mask wearing represented an undue burden, and that it was stigmatizing for healthcare workers since it identified them as people who hadn't been immunized. They also argued that the vaccine was "not effective enough" to be made a requirement—basing this on the ongoing scientific debate and the international call for better vaccines. And yet, despite the vocal protests of a few, with a strong effort at education and dramatically increased access to the vaccine across all settings, the immunization rates in healthcare workers in B.C. soared from an all-time low of only 30 percent in hospitals and 58 percent in care homes the year before the VOM policy to 80 percent in both settings the first year after.

The grievance hearing was held the following year, in 2013. I participated as an expert witness on three issues: the effectiveness and safety of vaccines, the implications of influenza on residents of long-term care and patients in hospital, and the rationale for the option of wearing a mask if a person wasn't immunized. The hearings over several weeks in July and September of 2013 were detailed and contentious, though respectful on all sides. The benefits, risks, and effectiveness of vaccines were thoroughly debated, and the wearing of masks as a method of "source control" of infected healthcare workers who may not yet have symptoms was deliberated at length.

The evidence on masks was scant and certainly not as well defined as that on immunization. But there was some evidence to show that masks can keep one's droplets in and prevent the infectious virus from escaping, and some evidence also to support the idea that healthcare workers who wear masks receive protection from patients, visitors, or residents who might be infected with influenza. Scientists who worked in laboratories testing and experimenting with masks and respirators (a type of mask designed to specifically filter out very small particles and that must be fit with a seal; the most common kind used in healthcare is the N95) made the case that in the laboratory there is leakage from surgical masks, which means both that a healthcare worker may not be protected from very small droplets from someone else and that these masks may not contain all their own expired droplets.

This contrasted with the evidence from infection prevention and control experts who work in hospital and long-term care settings, where use of masks has been shown to prevent transmission of influenza in a practical real-world environment. My role was to place the mask and the immunization discussion in the context of the broader influenza protection program that we believed was essential to preventing the introduction of this potentially lethal virus into the settings where people were most vulnerable. It meant that, along with the cornerstone practices of vaccination and mask wearing, we would have measures like rapid identification of ill patients and healthcare workers, meticulous hand hygiene and cough etiquette for all, restrictions on people working in or visiting places where outbreaks were happening, and use of antiviral medications.

Just as the 2013–2014 influenza season was ramping up and immunization programs were starting, we received the decision. On October 23, 2013, arbitrator Robert Diebolt, QC, released his 115-page award, wherein he found that the policy we had introduced in British Columbia was a "valid exercise of employer management rights." The grievance was dismissed. In summary, Diebolt believed the policy to be a valid and proportional response to improving the safety of all in healthcare settings. He commented as well that the policy provisions in his opinion did not breach the sections of the Charter of Rights and Freedoms the union had claimed. Although this was a definitive victory for the policy, by no means did it end the unions' concerns, and every year we continue to work to address these issues. These policies are always a balance between an individual's rights and the need to protect those we care for, in this case the more vulnerable residents and patients in our healthcare system. Public health considerations deal with complex ethical questions all the time, whether it's immunization to protect an individual and the community or notification of someone who's been exposed to a communicable disease. And we must find that fine balance between assiduously protecting individual privacy and making sure we can protect others from harm—a fine balance that's not always easy to find and hold.

ALTHOUGH THIS DISCUSSION OF POLICIES for the prevention of seasonal influenza may seem light years away from pandemic preparedness, in many ways our years dealing with such epidemics are relevant to a pandemic response. For those of us in public health, 2009 was a trial run that led us to rethink our plans. We realized that the pandemic phases the WHO had developed—imaginatively called phases 1 to 6—weren't readily understandable to most people and led to confusion. We also recognized that the phases were too broad, and that different areas of the world would be in different stages at the same time. And for large countries like Canada, the pandemic could hit very differently in different provinces, territories, and even communities. From the early onslaught in the province of B.C., both with the first wave in April and the second in September, to the differential impact on remote and northern communities and on Indigenous communities, pandemic influenza was a varied experience in many parts of the country. In addition, the ethical underpinnings of our responses were still not clearly articulated, and we needed to be very explicit on such important issues as who would get the vaccine first and how decisions would be made about access to such key resources as ventilators. We also needed more realistic scenarios to plan for generally.

In 2011, after the public inquiries and after-action reports were done and digested, I was asked to chair a national committee to deconstruct our Canadian Pandemic Influenza Plan, or CPIP (pronounced *c-pip*), as we affectionately called it. We started this work ostensibly as a two-year time-limited committee, with a mandate to develop realistic scenarios, review the evidence from and experience with the 2009 pandemic globally, and revise our CPIP accordingly.

Nine years later, as 2020 dawned, I was still chairing this committee and we were still working on the plan. Despite drastically reduced resources and waxing and waning political commitment in the interim, we'd made tremendous progress. Importantly, we had developed an updated "main body" to the plan that embedded ethical principles in all aspects of a pandemic response, contained realistic scenarios based on real-world experiences, and took into account the country's geographic and population differences.

We'd also completed and approved a number of key operational "annexes" to the main body of the plan, including ones on the availability of antivirals, laboratory testing, vaccines and immunization, and protocols for communications and surveillance. We were in the process of finishing our public health measures annex and had been working with colleagues globally on reviewing all the evidence for making decisions with great social impacts, such as closures of schools and businesses, international travel, social distancing, and mask wearing in the community.

Indeed, in the fall of 2019 I'd attended a workshop in Rome that had been arranged as part of the G7 commitment to developing a comprehensive pandemic influenza plan based on the best evidence we had collectively. The three-day workshop was stimulating and practical and gave us all an opportunity to review and understand detailed experiences from countries such as Japan and Italy along with the U.S., U.K., and Canada to large cities such as Hong Kong. We worked through the evidence for and experience of such measures as school closures, for example. (Were they able to stop or at least delay transmission? Did they have unintended negative consequences for children and families?) And what about closing businesses or prohibiting mass gatherings, from religious services to sports events? What were considered essential services? Were masks useful in the community? In retrospect, this occasion marked a culmination for me of several decades of thinking on these critical issues, gathered from my colleagues globally. Little did any of us know then that clouds were already forming, and that our seemingly abstract discussions would soon inform critical decisions around the world. Those lovely fall days walking through the bustling, ancient streets of Rome now seem surreal. Only a few short months later, those same streets would be deserted.

Looking back on it now, I think, How could we have known?

THE YEAR 2020 BEGAN in the same frenetic way that 2019 had ended. After the brief respite on the island of Barbados with my sister, I was thrown again into the fray on my first day back in the office. Burning anxiety in the pit of my stomach had become my constant companion—it was a feeling of dread, a feeling that things were happening in the world that we couldn't yet see, let alone control.

I also felt an intense and disturbing sense of déjà vu. China had begun reporting a "few" cases of "atypical pneumonia" in Wuhan, a city most Canadians had never heard of. *Serious respiratory infection, cause unknown.* Just as in 2003. Just as in SARS.

When it came to influenza and coronaviruses, China had some of the most knowledgeable scientists in the world—and in the past few years they'd reported diligently on new or variant strains that had arisen there and in the autonomous areas of Hong Kong and Taiwan. So why were they downplaying this one? If China, of all countries, couldn't diagnose this new virus as one of the known respiratory pathogens and were referring to it only as atypical pneumonia again, just as they had during SARS, this was cause for concern. It meant it was something new, possibly something that could be lethal and spread quickly: the most dangerous combination. Was this another failure of communication? As the days in January ticked along, my roiling sense of dread and déjà vu did not ease one bit.

And as it turned out, we were right to be concerned.

PART I

BE KIND

{ Week One: Before and After March 12 }

IN DR. BONNIE HENRY'S WORDS

On December 31, 2019, the Wuhan Municipal Health Commission in China's Hubei province issued a public statement:

> We have identified cases of pneumonia of unknown cause, associated with a local live seafood market.
>
> Chinese authorities report that there is no evidence of person-to-person spread at this time. The local live seafood market has been closed and a full investigation, including laboratory testing, of these cases is underway to identify the cause of the illness.
>
> While the cause of the illnesses in Wuhan, China, is still under investigation, SARS, avian and human influenza viruses, MERS-COV, adenovirus, and common respiratory pathogens have been ruled out. Pathogen identification and tracing of the cause is ongoing.

It was the first week of January when things truly began to speed up. Reports from China, coming through the informal online surveillance network, were increasingly worrisome. The first report had arrived in late December, when an ophthalmologist, Dr. Li, at Wuhan Central Hospital had posted on Weibo a warning to his fellow doctors. Beware of people with a "SARS-like" illness, his message said, and wear protective equipment. This doctor had seen seven cases in his clinic and knew there were others quarantined in his hospital.

At the same time, rumours were flying about vendors at the bustling Huanan Seafood Wholesale Market in Wuhan getting sick. At first the posts mentioned only those who worked at the market itself, but then, more ominously, word came that some of those affected were customers or family of the workers. These messages were translated and avidly followed by public health teams worldwide, including in Canada and in my own province, where the influenza team at the British Columbia Centre for Disease Control (BCCDC) tracked everything with keen interest. We knew there were strong links between our communities in B.C. and those across the Pacific Ocean, particularly in China, Hong Kong, and South Korea. And because we'd been hit by SARS twenty years before, we understood the potential impact here at home if these rumours were true. Our antennae were acutely attuned to all things respiratory in Asia.

I made my way back to my office in the province's capital city of Victoria that first Saturday in January, determined to review the posts again and connect with my colleagues at the BCCDC in Vancouver. Nothing was certain yet—some posts had been refuted and Dr. Li had been shut down—but the worry remained. Beijing was saying the outbreak was a small cluster, atypical pneumonia, linked to direct contact with animals at the market. Despite being called a seafood market, like most wet markets in China and throughout Asia, the market in Wuhan also had areas for produce, poultry, and other animals—including live animals that could be butchered on site. As well, in the back shadows if you knew where to look, there was illegal trading in exotic and wild animals, creatures like civet cats, which had been linked to the SARS virus, raccoon dogs, and pangolins.

On December 31 we'd released the first of what would become many alerts to our network in B.C.: to watch carefully for respiratory illness in people who may have travelled, to take precautions such as wearing masks and eye protection, and to isolate anyone sick as soon as possible. By our second alert, on January 3, the reported cases from Wuhan were up to forty-four, with eleven people in critical condition.

And then, on January 8, came word of fifty-nine cases and the news that we were dealing with a new coronavirus. It was news that heightened my anxiety and made my heart sink.

Like influenza, coronaviruses had been circling the globe for hundreds of years, but we'd known little about them until the 2003 SARS outbreak galvanized the virology world's attention. After SARS was pushed back into nature, researchers found that several viruses in the same family had been causing illness in humans, under the radar, for many years.

At first we simply lumped these in with all the other viruses that caused the "common cold," but once tests had been developed that gave us the means to look at the genetic material of viruses in minute detail, we recognized that these were different. Four coronaviruses were now known to cause illness: the first, OC43, had been around for decades and probably arose from cows that had in turn been infected by bats; this virus, though it caused mild disease today, was thought to have been the cause of a pandemic in 1890. The second, named 229E, had been around since the 1960s. And then there were two that had been identified since SARS: HKU1 and NL63.

What stymied researchers, though, was why some coronaviruses made that leap from animals to humans and produced only mild cold-like illness, whereas every now and then a strain emerged that wreaked havoc, like SARS and what became known as MERS (Middle Eastern Respiratory Syndrome). MERS also stems from a coronavirus, one that we now know is found in dromedary camels and occasionally spreads to humans who can then spread it to others, particularly when very sick and in hospital. The first major outbreak of this new coronavirus was detected in Saudi Arabia in 2012 and subsequently spread to a number of other countries, mostly in the Middle East. There was also a large outbreak in South Korea that sickened hundreds. The world went on alert when this new virus emerged; would this be the next pandemic? But despite giving rise to clusters of severe illness and deaths in healthcare settings, MERS did not spread widely, and outbreaks were detected and contained thanks to a concerted global effort led by the WHO. In January, this was a slight cause for hope.

WITHIN DAYS OF THE REPORT that a novel coronavirus had been detected in at least some people infected with this mysterious new illness, the genomic sequence of the virus was published on the international GenBank website. This boded well, since virus experts across the globe could now begin developing a test and then perhaps treatments or vaccines. It was a critical step, and reassuring: after China's secrecy in the first few weeks, its sharing of the genetic code for this new virus meant we were seeing a new openness, one we needed internationally in order to respond to this new threat.

Public health laboratories around the world, including the National Microbiology Lab in Winnipeg and the provincial Public Health Lab at the BCCDC, got to work. The medical microbiologists and virologists in these labs had been at the forefront of SARS, HINI, and Ebola, and had unparalleled expertise in developing new tests for just such pathogens.

I dared to breathe again. If we had a test, we would at least be light years ahead of the 2003 SARS outbreak, when we'd had no way to tell the difference between the new virus and all the other causes of cough and fevers in a northern winter.

Still, watching events unfold in Wuhan through the veil of official reports—and the often contradictory but frightening virtual reports that leaked through—had all of us in public health on edge. The public health leaders from the provinces and territories, as well as from the federal Public Health Agency of Canada, started to talk more frequently, adding the new coronavirus to our agenda. We were a mix of new faces alongside some of us who had lived through past crises from SARS to HINI to Ebola—and for me and others in the latter category, these past experiences made us more wary and worried. Increasingly, we directed the conversations towards the need to quickly step up our preparedness. The same thing was happening in countries around the world and at the WHO: leaders and experts were pulling together to watch, to share, and to prepare.

I was chair of the Council of Chief Medical Officers of Health (CCMOH), made up of the senior public health doctors in each province and territory as well as nationally. Its purpose is to share, coordinate, and advocate for health promotion and protection in the country—and, when circumstances require it, to morph into the lead body providing public health advice in an emergency. Back in 2003, when SARS hit, Canada had neither a council of medical officers nor a public health agency, and our national response, as critiqued in all the ensuing inquiries, was wanting because of it. As a result, the Public Health Agency of Canada (PHAC) was created to be the federal agency to lead the important surveillance and health protection roles, separate from the machinery of government; it would speak to the public directly and advise the government independently on health matters. CCMOH and PHAC had already been called into action in 2009 for the H1N1 pandemic, and the response, while by no means perfect, was exponentially better than our national response had been during SARS.

As we watched the happenings in China closely, seeing hospitals in the city of Wuhan fill up as neighbourhoods were locked down, our agenda became increasingly focused on this new coronavirus. We knew there were no direct flights to Canada from Wuhan, but there were many, many flights from other cities in China. They came directly to three airports in Canada: Montreal, Toronto, and Vancouver. Thousands of passengers a day arrived from the world's most populous country—not to mention the thousands more who came indirectly through Seoul, Hong Kong, and Taiwan, or through Los Angeles, Chicago, and New York. Advisories were issued against travel to Wuhan and Hubei province, but tracking the tens of thousands coming in through more indirect routes seemed an impossible task.

In B.C., as in every other province, we understood that our health systems would be the ones affected, and that our public health teams in regions and communities across the province would be the first line of protection. And so, as we do for every concerning illness that may be transmitted between people, public health officials stepped up surveillance and case detection.

This meant closely monitoring our influenza-like illness (ILI) surveillance in our labs, physicians' offices, and hospitals for any indication of a surge that could be connected to this new virus. It was influenza season in Canada, and we were seeing lots of illness—mostly influenza A H3N2 in older people and a smattering of influenza A HINI in younger adults, as well as the myriad other respiratory viruses that cause everything from severe infections to the common cold. These were viruses like RSV (respiratory syncytial virus), parainfluenza, enterovirus, and rhinoviruses. We were also seeing already known coronaviruses, ones that cause mild colds in most people, with occasional outbreaks of moderate illness in long-term care homes.

IN LATE JANUARY 2020, our hospitals in Canada were experiencing the typical winter surge of older people being admitted for pneumonias—and also for exacerbations of other conditions, such as heart disease and lung disease, that inevitably follow influenza infection. As was normal for this time of year, hospitals were running full, and emergency departments were at capacity dealing with the daily flow of trauma and disease; ILI surveillance in doctors' offices showed that our community illness was in the 90 percent range, signalling the peak of our influenza season. And it was in this haystack of respiratory illness that we needed to be on guard for a single case of the new respiratory illness, the proverbial needle, and to ensure that the case was isolated, the patient cared for safely, and transmission prevented.

Within ten days of the genome sequence being published, the public health lab at the BCCDC, working around the clock and using the technology and expertise they had honed in-house on influenza and other virus tests, had developed a test that could identify this novel coronavirus—provisional and yet to be fully validated, but at least it gave us a chance of finding someone with this troubling new virus. And as it turned out, not a moment too soon. Meanwhile, my own focus was on rallying not only the public health teams but also the entire health system for readiness.

I was just two years into my role as provincial health officer for B.C., taking over after the retirement of the beloved and universally respected Dr. Perry Kendall, my mentor and dear friend, who'd been in the role for almost twenty years. My relationship with Adrian Dix, the minister of health, reflected this newness. He, too, had taken on his role recently, only a few months before me, when his party had won a minority government. And now here we were, thrust into the middle of what could be the biggest challenge in our lifetime, with only the beginnings of the trust and shared experience in dealing with issues that are requisite for a functional relationship. So much depended on us getting it right.

I'd notified the minister early in January, as soon as we began hearing about the illness in Wuhan, and had been providing short updates through the ensuing weeks. By the middle of January the press were also starting to call me, wanting my take on what was happening around the world and what might happen here. Indeed, in one early interview I declared that, given our travel patterns and connections with China, I fully expected we would have cases in B.C. Alarmingly, this made the front page of our national newspaper at a time when most messages from across Canada were much more cautious and reassuring.

Just like every other chief medical officer of health across the country, I had a mandate and the legal authority to speak directly to the public about issues related to health. I was fully aware, however, that if I were wildly offside with what the provincial health minister and government believed, it could make my position challenging, and that if I was too far off the mark too often, the government could render me ineffective or fire me altogether. It's a fine balance—to be effective in the protection of the public's health and to promote that larger goal in a way that engages without alienating. Or, as my mentor often said in reference to the challenge and delicacy of this role, "You can make a point or you can make a difference." What this meant in practice was that, as much as we may wish to, we didn't have to immediately take on the cause of every injustice or health inequity . . . at least, not right away.

For many issues in public health, knowing when to push—and when to keep the solution in your back pocket until the right political and societal moment arises—is a skill. And for public health leaders everywhere, it's the fundamental challenge: we want to make change for the sake of health but must also be sensitive to the many fiscal and political realities that exist in a democracy.

When I publicly expressed my informed belief that we'd likely see cases of this new coronavirus in B.C., I hit a nerve with the minister. But this gave me an opportunity to talk with him, and with our deputy minister of health, about why I was so sure and what else, realistically, I could see potentially happening here. I knew it was critically important for us to be forthright and open, even when the news was bad, in order to build trust with the people we served. My work in Pakistan with polio, in Uganda with the dreaded Ebola virus, and in Toronto with SARS had led me to believe deeply that telling people the realistic worst and preparing them for it was not only right, but necessary. Time and again we've seen that during a crisis people will do the right thing, that they'll be overwhelmingly altruistic and kind—if we prepare them as best we can, inform them of the right thing to do, and give them the means to do it. We saw this in New York City on 9/11, in New Orleans during the aftermath of Katrina, and in countless other disasters around the globe. But, of course, this isn't always the natural inclination for governments and political leaders, for whom bad news can be a political nightmare.

More and more I was coming to accept that this new virus in China was going to find its way here, and probably before too long. Looking back, though, I hadn't yet realized that it would traverse the globe in quite the destructive way it eventually did.

All too soon, what I had foreshadowed became reality.

BY THE THIRD WEEK of January, the WHO was holding daily or near-daily briefings. We in the public health community watched as cases in China climbed, first to hundreds, then thousands, then suddenly tens of thousands. The movement of people for the Lunar New Year celebrations had led to a spread of the virus across much of the country, and by February the central government was responding in earnest. We looked on agog as a thousand-bed isolation hospital was built in days in Wuhan, and as the hospital system in that huge metropolis became whelmed then overwhelmed. Strict lockdown measures were imposed on the city's almost twelve million people, restricting everyone to their homes, stopping bus and train service, and establishing roadblocks to prevent travel into or out of Wuhan. Ground zero was walled off—or so it was hoped.

We in Canada, in step with countries around the world, issued more travel advisories for the province of Hubei. In retrospect, of course, this was like putting a tiny bandage on a hemorrhaging artery. Thousands of people a day continued to enter our country from other cities in China and to move around the globe. The idea that we could stop this routine air travel between nations on a global scale wasn't something that anyone, or any country, had yet seriously considered.

Instead we were still in the influenza mindset, one in which travel restrictions are futile, given the nature of influenza with its impossibly short incubation period—just one to three days—and the fact that it spread before people were aware they were infected. And travel bans could be destructive by blocking access to foods, medicines, and other essentials that countries rely upon. Even in retrospect, though, it's hard to know what we could have done to stop the movement of the virus in those early days. Countries that had put stringent travel restrictions in place early on, such as the United States and Italy, were hit just as hard as those that had been more open and watchful. What we did know was that our public health teams had to be ready to detect and contain rapidly as we prepared for the worst.

In B.C., we started testing people who had returned from travel—with our new BCCDC-developed test—by the third week of January. With limited test capacity, however, we asked clinicians across the province to focus on travellers with the symptoms we knew were associated with this novel corona-virus. Alerts went out daily to emergency departments and community physicians with the latest updates on where the virus had been detected: from Wuhan, Hubei, to other cities and provinces of China, and from Hong Kong to Singapore and Korea. We also gave clinicians licence to test anyone they were concerned about, even if they hadn't travelled to known risk areas. This was a safety net, a way of making sure that if someone had had contact with a sick person, they, too, would be tested. We wanted our so-called index of suspicion to be high; this virus was moving, and we needed to stay ahead of it as best we could.

OUR FIRST CASE CAME sooner than any of us had imagined. A Vancouver man who'd travelled to Wuhan for work developed the classic symptoms: cough, headache, fever. His wife, who'd been reading about the new virus, had insisted that upon his return he shelter in their home, wear a mask at all times, and stay away from her and their young child. When the man's symptoms began, the couple went directly to the local emergency, where they were quickly isolated and tested. I got the call from the lab on a Sunday morning: they'd run it twice using three different markers on the virus RNA and would be sending it to the National Microbiology Lab in Winnipeg for confirmation, but given the travel history and the results from our test, they were confident it was a true positive. We swiftly arranged a teleconference huddle with the provincial lab, the local medical officer of health, and the emergency physician who'd seen the case in order to coordinate our plan. Although we already had a protocol in place, we knew the response to our first detection would be essential to get right, in every detail.

Only the day before, on January 25, the first case in Canada, in another province, had been announced publicly. The press conference that followed, with six different spokespeople, had not gone as well as planned. I knew that, in order to allay the fear building in our communities in B.C., we needed to be open and clear and to show that we were managing this new threat in the best possible way. And it wasn't only fear: an irrational backlash against the Asian community was starting to happen, with racial attacks on Chinese and other Asian people, and on businesses in the Asian community, being reported with increasing frequency.

The health minister and I had talked about our approach and agreed it would be just the two of us delivering the news; we also agreed to be the consistent voice of the team supporting us, in both public health and government, as we faced this new threat. We'd already planned to deliver our first live media brief the following day, a Monday, to discuss the initiatives underway in our healthcare system and in the provincial lab and within public health. Now we'd be announcing that the novel coronavirus itself had indeed arrived on our shores.

I flew to Vancouver early in the morning, watching the sun rise over the mountains and wondering what the coming days would bring. Was this the start of a flood of cases, or would we be able to contain the virus, at least for a time? From past experience with crises, I knew that much would depend on my ability to get the information people needed out there in a way that conveyed the risk and the uncertainty while showing that we had plans in place and that there were things each of us could do to protect ourselves and our families.

I also knew how critical it was to protect the confidentiality of the case—the man we'd labelled "BC1." My experience with SARS and Ebola had made this very clear to me: although baseless, there's a stigma against people who develop a new, potentially deadly disease, and if they're publicly identified they can be subjected to threats and harassment by media and even by their own community. This had happened in the remote community of Gulu in Northern Uganda, where the huts of families with Ebola cases had been burned to the ground. But this kind of reaction wasn't unique to that country, nor to the disease of Ebola. In Toronto during the SARS outbreak, citizens of Chinese background had been vilified despite the fact that SARS had affected people across all ethnic racial backgrounds and socio-economic strata. The families of some of the cases had been hounded relentlessly by media who were trying to get ever more information on those who were ill. In one particularly egregious case, the teenage son of a person who'd died from SARS had been tracked down at home and ambushed as he prepared to leave for his mother's funeral.

This type of behaviour not only has serious effects on those families who are trying to manage the shock and tragedy of having a new, frightening illness in their midst; it also makes others who may have symptoms reluctant to come forward for testing and care. Our ability in public health to find cases, to ensure they receive the care they need, and to protect families and the community is seriously undermined if people believe they will be identified publicly. In my role managing the 2003 outbreak, I'd talked with every family who'd lost someone to SARS. I'd witnessed the pain they suffered and seen how it was made so much more acute by public fear and reaction. I was determined not to let that happen again with this new coronavirus.

Our first press briefing was held at the B.C. Centre for Disease Control in Vancouver—a way to highlight the important work the BCCDC was doing in developing our tests as well as coordinating the lab response and, in concert with my office, the public health response. It was the first press briefing the minister and I had done together, and I was more than a little nervous. We'd spent several hours with key leaders from the BCCDC and the health system working through the details of what we would present: coronavirus 101; an update on what we knew from China; what the WHO was saying; the lab testing we were doing; and the details the public needed to know about the first case. We had agreed to release only what was needed, and at a level of detail that couldn't be personally identifiable: a returning traveller, a man in his fifties who lived in the Vancouver Coastal Health region. We'd let people know that a small number of close contacts were being monitored and that the man himself was being monitored in isolation at home (importantly, not in hospital). I also notified Canada's chief public health officer, my colleague Dr. Theresa Tam, as was our protocol. This notification was passed from her and the Public Health Agency to the WHO, fulfilling our obligation under the IHR. Then it was time for the minister and me to go.

The large conference room in the basement of the BCCDC was packed with lights and cameras and reporters from all the local and national TV, radio, and print outlets. I took a deep breath and tried to suppress the panic I was feeling. Minister Dix spoke first, with introductions, and then I was on.

It was almost two hours later before we'd exhausted all the reporters' questions. Inevitably, there was a push for more details. Why would we not release the exact age and place where the person lived? Why would we not say what hospital they'd gone to? Why release information by regional health authority only—wasn't that too large an area? How many people were being tested, how many tests were pending, how sure were we that the test was right, how long would it take to confirm? And there were many, many questions about the virus itself—at that time still saddled with the ungainly moniker "novel coronavirus": how was it transmitted, who was at risk, what could we do, what did we know about what was actually happening in China?

Much of our advice was simple, but what we knew worked: wash your hands regularly, cover your mouth when you cough, stay away from others if you're sick and if you've travelled to areas where the novel coronavirus was circulating, call ahead so you could be tested safely. We'd also set up our provincial "nurse line," 811, for people to call to have their symptoms assessed. Because this was a coronavirus, it was spread between people through respiratory droplets that are inhaled into the nasal passages or lungs, and we suspected that, like many other respiratory viruses, it could last in droplets on surfaces for a time. As a result, urging people to clean their hands before touching their face, eyes, or mouth was also vitally important. These were our first messages—and even with all we've learned about the virus since, this advice remains the cornerstone of how we protect ourselves and others.

BEHIND THE SCENES in the health system, we were making radical changes to prepare for the possibility that this novel coronavirus could take off in our province. We set up a provincial health emergency response committee that would report to the deputy minister and me. It would be a single coordinating body for the entire health system, from long-term care to hospitals to public health. This meant we could assess our human resource needs as well as our needs for such critical items as personal protective equipment (PPE: gloves, gowns, masks, and respirators), ventilators, ECMO (extracorporeal membrane oxygenation) machines, acute care and ICU beds, and lab capacity ranging from reagents to swabs to technicians. The idea was to be able to shift people and resources around if and when required.

At our first meetings, it became clear that it would take

some effort to get everyone aligned; it was also clear that our PPE stockpile had been eroded in the years since the 2009 pandemic and would need considerable work to build back up. In this we were not alone. Already we were hearing from China and around the world that there were delays and challenges in obtaining masks and the widely used N95 respirators in particular, not to mention ventilators. As we watched the outbreak in Wuhan expand logarithmically, and hospitals become full with the ill, stories also surfaced, through the informal channels of healthcare workers, about people not being able to get the masks and face shields and gowns they needed to safely care for patients. Healthcare workers were getting sick, and the critical care beds and ventilators needed to keep people breathing through the severe lung infections the virus caused were in short supply. Exacerbating the situation was the fact that much of the world relied on the cheap manufacturing in China for their supplies of these critical items, and much of that was centred in Hubei province, in and around Wuhan. As people fell sick, that critical manufacturing was being shut down, and workers either became ill themselves or were sent home to isolate. And so, as we reorganized our healthcare system to prepare ourselves, the work of obtaining the PPE we needed became of paramount importance. Step one was to develop a database of exactly what we had where, and then project what the need might be. For this we turned to modelling.

We had a history of using modelling to help us understand the scenarios we might face in a crisis just like this one. In 2009, modellers at the BCCDC were able to give us advice on the best immunization strategies for protecting as many people as possible in the most efficient way. I'd been working with modellers for many years and knew how valuable their input could be, but I was also well aware of the dangers of using models, given that so many people believed they could predict the future. As we often said among ourselves in this sphere, "All models are wrong; some are useful." Models are all dependent on the inputs, or "parameters," that are entered into complex computer simulations; parameters might include incubation period, number of contacts, probability of needing hospitalization, and probability of needing ICU care. I knew that the closer we in public health connected with our modellers, the better they would understand the range of possibilities for each parameter, and the more useful the model would be.

Luckily, we had integrated senior scientists with expertise in modelling into the BCCDC several years before. Now they were tasked with helping support our preparedness for and response to this new coronavirus. Their work would prove invaluable.

The approach we took deviated from that of other groups internationally and across Canada. Initially, we focused on those areas of the world that were experiencing exponential growth in the virus and analyzed their parameters; we then applied those to the situation in B.C. This helped us develop realistic estimates of how many people we might see who needed to be in hospital and more specifically in the ICU. We could then adjust our health services and the attendant PPE to meet those needs. Still, as we soon realized, none of this was simple—and as this virus, now named COVID-19, escaped its origins and affected countries in Europe, these models took on almost epic importance.

THE SECOND CASE DETECTED in the province followed rapidly on the heels of BC1, except that this time it was a person who hadn't travelled. At our case huddle, the spectre that this might be a locally acquired case gave us all pause. But public health teams went to work and soon determined that although the case, BC2, hadn't travelled, she had received family visitors in the days before she became ill, and they had come from Wuhan. The teams went to her house and interviewed each household member, taking swabs to test everyone and hoping we might be able to identify someone who'd brought this virus with them from elsewhere. The other possibility—that the patient had acquired the virus locally, indicating that at this early stage it was already in our community—was a frightening scenario we all hoped wasn't so. But within days two of the family members also tested positive, both with mild disease. There were a few more contacts to follow up with this time, but all were isolated and monitored for the incubation period— which, to the best of our knowledge, was fourteen days—and none of them became ill.

As we moved through February, this soon became our routine: a case huddle, a public health investigation, monitoring of contacts, and supporting people who were ill. Most could be cared for at home, although several needed short stays in hospital. We were also learning more and more about COVID-19 and the virus that caused it—now named SARS coronavirus-2. Among my direct team and contacts, only a few of us had weathered the storm that was SARS in 2003—and for me, the very name, SARS-2, triggered the memories and anxieties that had taken over our lives almost seventeen years before.

For the newer public health experts, I knew, this seemed strange. When I insisted on following up every contact and requiring these people to isolate at home, I got some pushback; this was much more than we usually did when people were contacts of those infected with other diseases like measles or even TB. Part of me worried that my own traumatic memories were making me overreact, but still I explained to our teams, over and over, that this was different, this was potentially devastating, and yes, we did need to take these seemingly draconian measures. And so, although not perhaps fully on board, the public health teams did as I asked as more and more cases came to light. After one particularly challenging discussion, one of my colleagues, who'd been suggesting we were overreacting, responded to my direction with "As you wish."

"Does that make me Princess Buttercup?" I responded. Not everyone got the reference, but it did cut the tension and we acknowledged that we were all in this together.

By February, public health teams were managing every case. Contacts were being tracked and isolated, and we were finding infected people across the province—from the Lower Mainland, where most of the population and most of the cases arose, to the Interior and Vancouver Island. So far, the more remote and underserved communities in the north were relatively protected. But since we knew that the potential impact could be much greater and more worrisome if cases arose there, much of our health system planning focused on supporting these communities, many of which are Indigenous. We were keenly aware that the history of pandemics had not been kind to First Nations— and indeed in some cases had devastated nations—so we were determined that it would be different this time. Early on, we engaged with the First Nations Health Authority and with Indigenous communities to try to make sure they were integrated into our response and preparations.

Our mantra remained "contain, delay, prepare." The preparation part of that motto was the purview of the deputy minister of health. Our respective teams had worked through the possible and probable scenarios together, using all the data and information we could find from those countries that were now being tested with the onslaught of COVID-19. We started with all we knew from Wuhan and Hubei, and then with what we were unexpectedly seeing unfold before us in Northern Italy.

The tragedy in Italy had taken the world by surprise—suddenly there were hundreds of cases, then thousands; hospitals were full, then overfull. The trauma of having to make decisions about who would get access to the scarce ventilators was painful to hear about. Doctors and nurses were falling ill, some dying; others were left traumatized by not being able to care for their fellow citizens as the virus raged through their communities. We were unwilling voyeurs helplessly watching the trauma unfold a continent away while knowing it could well play out here, too: that we, too, could be faced with the same impossible decisions of who would get the last ventilator, or how to make the limited masks last the shift, or who would be there to hold the hand of a dying person. While many of us who watched respiratory viruses, and had planned for pandemics for decades, had held out hope that China could control this new threat, what took place in Italy made us realize that this was not to be. We now understood that we needed to be ready, all of us everywhere. The virus was coming.

AS WE IN THE PROVINCES and territories of Canada prepared to protect our health systems and avoid the scenarios we were seeing in Wuhan and more recently Italy, the federal government was looking outward to support Canadians who'd been stranded in Hubei. Other countries had been doing the same, getting their citizens out as lockdowns became more extreme and access to care more tenuous. As February progressed this international rescue mission became a singular focus of the federal government. In retrospect, we can see that it may have taxed our expertise at that level and turned attention away from the issues that were building domestically—issues that would soon come to define our response to the pandemic in Canada. But in February, perhaps we still had hope that the virus wouldn't spread as widely—after all, the WHO still hadn't declared a pandemic. So, we in Canada added repatriation to our response lexicon and worked together to get our citizens home.

The first suggestion was that Canadians returning from abroad should come to Vancouver, but we in B.C. quickly responded that this wasn't a viable option. On our many calls with the federal teams, we were able to make it clear that the airport at YVR was in the middle of an urban environment, that there was no way to limit access to the press and others, and that, most urgently, there were no readily available accommodations to keep people for the mandatory fourteen-day quarantine period. Early in the discussion about where to send people I'd suggested that Trenton, in Ontario, might be a possibility; it was, as I knew from my previous life as a physician in the Canadian military, an expansive air force base with ample runway room and accommodations designed to house the many international air force personnel who came to Canada for training.

Eventually Trenton was the anointed destination, but flights would need to land at YVR for refuelling. Planes were found and the mission began in the early hours of February 6. Politics and weather delays caused several sleepless nights for the teams in the air and on the ground. Finally more than

300 Canadians were on-board and headed home. Our emergency response team set up shop at YVR: it was intended as a short refuelling stop, but we had to be prepared for other possibilities. If anyone developed symptoms on the thirteen-hour flight to Vancouver, they'd be taken off the plane, assessed, and potentially quarantined here. So, just in case, we had the hospital on standby, the staff briefed, and a hotel at the ready. That had been its own small drama, as we took over an isolated wing of a hotel across the street from the designated hospital near the airport. The hotel, perhaps understandably, was not at all pleased when we showed up with an order from the federal quarantine service. They soon realized, however, that this was not something they should fight, and all safety measures would be put in place to ensure staff were protected—and, of course, it would all be paid for.

It was late in the evening when we received word that our planes in China had been granted airspace and were allowed to take off; all passengers had been assessed multiple times and, so far, no one had fevers or symptoms. We heaved a sigh of relief and then hunkered down to wait. The first flight, Canada 1, arrived shortly after midnight; word from the tarmac came: "All is well." The flight took off again an hour later and landed safely in Trenton in the early morning. Canada 2 came through a few hours after that, and again it flew off without a hitch. There had been a few long, anxious nights for the team, but we were happy and proud: hundreds of stranded Canadians and their families had made it home.

AS FEBRUARY PROGRESSED, our approach—testing as widely as we could, managing every case in detail, finding contacts and isolating them so that if they did become ill, they would not pass this new virus on to others—seemed to be succeeding. This work, known as case management and contact tracing, is the bread and butter of public health, but it's also time-consuming and challenging, particularly when time is of the essence. Within hours of a positive test coming back, we would contact that person, find anyone with whom they'd been in close contact while they were infectious, and make sure we could isolate them. There was nothing we could do to prevent infection once someone had been exposed to the virus, so we had to go back to basics: keeping sick people away from well people and isolating those exposed for the incubation period. This was how we could break those chains of transmission and prevent the virus from causing rapidly growing outbreaks that would overwhelm our health system.

At the same time, we were learning more and more about COVID-19 and the virus that caused it: we found, for example, that the incubation period was holding firm at fourteen days, with most people developing symptoms around days five to seven. This meant it was a disease amenable to public health interventions like contact tracing—which was very different from influenza, for example, where the incubation period was three days at most, and people could pass the virus on to others before they showed symptoms themselves. We were also learning that COVID-19 was most severe in older people, especially those over seventy, and that, relatively speaking, children seemed to be spared from both infection and severe illness. There were theories as to why this might be, from lack of contact with others, given that schools had been closed, or lack of testing, to a paucity of receptors in younger people to which the virus binds. In short, we did not know then if this was merely an artifact or if it was real.

There were so many things we didn't know for sure. Could people pass the virus on before they had symptoms? And could people be infected, and be infectious to others, without showing any symptoms at all? There were stories coming out of China and Singapore, and soon from Italy, that suggested this might be the case—but it still didn't appear to be the main way the virus travelled. It was becoming clear that this was a virus that had adapted to humans and now spread between us with relative ease, but that it was also unique, not the same as other viruses we knew. It wasn't as infectious as influenza, for example, but it caused more severe illness, especially in older people; meanwhile it was more infectious than SARS but not as severe. This new virus, it turned out, had found a niche that put it into our most challenging pandemic scenario: it could spread easily in people who had minimal symptoms and might not even realize they were infected, and it could cause severe illness requiring hospitalization and ICU care in large numbers.

The minister and I were holding daily press briefings now, relaying what we knew to the public and providing updates on the cases here in B.C. These briefings became sometimes lengthy events as we attempted to answer all the new questions coming up. And it meant even longer days for me, since I needed to be not only on top of all the issues arising in B.C. but also on top of the latest data and information from around the world. Along with that, my colleagues and I across the country were having national Special Advisory Committee (SAC) calls, sometimes daily, and I was connecting regularly with a team at the WHO dedicated to policy around mass gatherings (usually at four a.m. my time, or afternoon in Geneva) and with my counterparts in Washington State, Oregon, Alaska, and Idaho—or "Region X," as that federal region is known in the United States.

———

FEBRUARY 20 WAS THE next day to be seared in my memory. Midway through that morning I received a call from the lab: we had another positive case, but this time the only travel had been to Iran.

Iran!? We were all shocked. Iran hadn't reported having any cases, but we knew that information coming out of the country was limited. The relationship between Canada and Iran had been strained for a long time, and had recently broken further after the shooting down in Tehran of a passenger airplane carrying 169 people, two-thirds of whom were Canadian or had ties to Canada. My first thought was that this must be a false positive or a contamination—or perhaps even a MERS infection that had cross-reacted. But the lab had already considered these possibilities and tested for MERS as well as for the other circulating coronaviruses. The results came back negative, even while the sample was COVID-19 positive on all three markers, and with a low cycle threshold (meaning lots of virus). The lab also sent the sample for whole-genome sequencing to determine whether it was the same as the viruses we'd seen in people who'd been in Wuhan—or different enough that it would help us understand how long it had been circulating in Iran. We were learning that this virus mutated slowly, but that over time even small changes in the RNA as it passed from person to person allowed us to track its movement. The genome results came through in hours: this strain of the new virus was indeed different from those we'd seen here before.

This was what's known in public health as a sentinel event: an important marker that the virus had spread more widely than we knew globally, and also an indicator that its spread in

Iran was happening on a large scale. As our public health teams sprang to work investigating the story of this new case, I reported these concerning new findings to our country's chief public health officer as well as the Public Health Agency of Canada, who urgently passed it on to the WHO.

Our press briefing that day was longer than usual as I explained the significance of this sentinel event. There were, understandably, many questions, but one was paramount: Why had the person been tested in the first place? Given our limited testing capacity, like our colleagues across the country we'd given priority to those with known risks for COVID-19—people who'd travelled to areas where we knew the virus was circulating or who'd had contact with someone who had travelled and was ill. Iran was not one of those areas. The woman who tested positive had visited family there during the New Year celebrations and then flown home through Tehran to Istanbul to Frankfurt. She'd become ill with an influenza-like illness several days after her return home to B.C. and was sick enough that she went to the local emergency department to be assessed. The doctor who saw her was initially sure she had influenza, but because she'd travelled on so many flights, and almost as an afterthought, had asked for a COVID-19 test as well. In short, we'd picked up the case partly through luck and partly thanks to our preparedness messaging: we'd told clinicians to maintain a low index of suspicion and to test if they believed the virus was at all a possibility. To paraphrase Louis Pasteur, luck favours the prepared.

AS FEBRUARY SLIPPED INTO MARCH we saw more and more cases, and in areas outside the populous Lower Mainland, but so far we'd contained transmission and found contacts before they could pass on the virus. Still, containment was becoming increasingly challenging, given the tens of thousands of people who were coming across our borders daily. We were also closely watching what was happening in the United States, where the reported virus activity was suspiciously low. President Trump's rhetoric—referring to the "China virus" as he imposed early travel restrictions on that nation, relying on these to stop importation—hadn't been helping; nor had his vitriolic criticisms of the WHO. My Region X colleagues told me they were worried: their country's acclaimed Centers for Disease Control and Prevention (CDC) had developed a test for the new virus but hadn't allowed individual states to develop their own. There had also been problems with the tests sent out from the CDC. This meant that only limited testing was available at the state level, and that local public health authorities needed to get permission for each test and then send the sample to the CDC in Atlanta. Several importations had been caught at the borders, but without testing available in hospitals and clinics for those with severe illness, my American colleagues were concerned that cases would be missed.

In B.C. we were beginning to reach the limits of our public health capacity and had begun reassigning staff from other critical functions to support our case finding and contact tracing. The virus, we knew, was on the move, with cases now in many European countries, particularly Italy, France, and Spain. A WHO investigation had confirmed that a large outbreak was ongoing in Iran after the case we'd detected. It was time for us to shift from a health system response to a full-government response. Seeing what was happening in China, and then what had happened in other affected countries, we knew that if we started experiencing community spread we'd need to coordinate action across every sector of our communities, from schools to universities to workplaces, and that we'd need the ability to define and protect our essential services—everything from food to transportation to health services. Already we were seeing a rise in anxiety levels, with people stocking up on essential items like canned food, masks, hand sanitizer, and, inexplicably, toilet paper.

My colleagues and I developed an expanded B.C. COVID-19 Pandemic Response Plan. Then, in the first week of March, the health minister, deputy minister, and I met with Premier John Horgan's office and cabinet to walk them through possible scenarios and potential challenges. It was a sobering presentation, made all the more real by events unfolding around the world: the dramatic images of hospitals being overwhelmed, whole cities in lockdown, people dying from COVID-19 and from lack of access to care for other health issues. And, of course, just as devastating as the immediate health impacts were the potential economic impacts.

On Thursday, March 5, at our press briefing in Vancouver, I announced eight new cases, including our first "community case": someone who had acquired their illness here in B.C. It represented the concerning next step in this emergency—one that we'd been expecting and preparing for while hoping against hope it wouldn't happen. The next day we held a technical briefing on the situation and our "whole of government" response plans with media and with each of the opposition parties. After that came the first media briefing in which the premier, the health minister, and I together told the public what we were planning and how we'd be responding. With COVID-19 moving so rapidly around the world, it was inevitable that it would take hold here, we said, but it was in our hands now to minimize the impact on our communities, our families, our loved ones.

Back at my Vancouver hotel that night, I slept fitfully. The many long days were catching up with me, but I could foresee many more ahead. Memories of the anxieties and fears, the sadness, anger, and grief we'd faced during the SARS outbreak came flooding back. I didn't know if I could do this again; it was going to be so hard for so many. Already we were seeing people react with anger and lashing out at "others"; already healthcare workers were afraid to go to work and demanding access to levels of PPE that were in short supply around the world.

The next morning's news did nothing to assuage my angst. Cases had been confirmed in a long-term care home. This was indeed the worst-case scenario all of us were dreading, knowing the deadly effect of this virus on our seniors and elders, particularly in a setting like long-term care. It was truly upon us now. I knew in my heart that the next few months would stretch us to our limits.

In our daily press briefing that Saturday, these thoughts overwhelmed me as I announced the outbreak at the Lynn Valley Care Centre. I fought back tears as my voice quivered with emotion, and I stopped to collect myself. I was concerned that breaking down in such a public way would scare people and only make the situation worse. When asked why I'd become emotional in the question-and-answer period afterwards, I explained how I knew we were heading for a difficult time and how we needed to support each other to get through it. Kindness and compassion, understanding others' suffering, would be the best way we could weather what was coming and avoid the trauma I'd seen in past crises.

———

THE FOLLOWING WEEK was the turning point; we fully entered the next phase of this crisis. Monday started with the first death of a resident in one of our long-term care homes. Then came reports from colleagues in Washington State that a new case had been detected—but possibly one that was related to the first case they'd found several weeks before. This meant that the virus had been circulating silently, and that potentially hundreds of people with COVID-19 were already in the community. They were investigating outbreaks in several elder-care homes that had been thought to be influenza, but now, in a much more concerning development, were likely COVID-19. Our borders with the U.S. were still wide open, and although we had advised people to limit travel, thousands were still crossing back and forth every day to see family and friends, to shop, to attend events. B.C. residents had always been very connected to our neighbours in the region known as Cascadia to the south, many identifying more closely with them than with our Canadian neighbours across the Rocky Mountains. As our community cases increased, more of the infected people were identifying travel or connection with Washington State as their only risk factor; we were also seeing people test positive who had travelled to many countries in the world that hadn't yet officially reported any cases. These included returning travellers from Egypt, India, and Russia, and from cruise ships in every ocean.

On our SAC calls that week, I heard the same story from my counterparts across the country: the WHO hadn't yet declared the outbreak to be a pandemic, but what we were seeing surely meant it was only a matter of time. This virus moved between people, and as a result it, like humans, was moving fast around the globe.

We were also seeing the virus spread in crowds, especially during what we called mass gatherings, which included everything from religious events to sports events to conferences—any place where people came together from disparate locations and connected, often inside "closed" environments, sharing food and drink and air space. We'd already put restrictions in place for these events, conveying urgent messages about hand hygiene, staying away if you were sick, not sharing food, and taking the names of attendees so that people could be contacted if needed. This was the protocol we'd developed over years of preparation for influenza pandemics, but it was becoming clear that it wasn't enough for this new virus; crowds with random mixing were the perfect way for COVID-19 to spread.

Knowing the risks and the potential impact of an outbreak if it happened during a medical conference, I had directed that several large meetings and conferences be postponed or cancelled. Unbeknownst to me, however, a big international dental conference in Vancouver had gone ahead in early March, with fourteen thousand dental professionals from around the world. On March 10 I was notified that someone who'd attended the conference had tested positive. They'd been at the conference for at least two hours during a window when they were infectious. My team and I thought this was a relatively low-risk exposure and opted to send out a notification publicly to warn people to check for symptoms. In the next two days, however, six more people in B.C. alone tested positive, and each one had been at the conference. We were hearing of cases in other provinces as well.

By Thursday, March 12, all these pieces were swirling in my

head. Critically, B.C.'s schools would begin their March break the next day. I knew that many families had plans to travel for the two-week holiday to countries all over the world, and that many cross-border events had been planned, particularly in Washington State. Canada had advised against travel to China and areas with known COVID-19 outbreaks but had resisted broader warnings than that. It seemed incomprehensible and impossible to shut borders with the U.S. in particular.

I was chairing our SAC calls that week. On March 12 we focused solely on two questions: What were we going to do about travel? And about mass gathering limitations? Although the details varied among provinces and regions, it was clear that we all believed we were at the point when we needed to take decisive action. Quebec, in particular, had been seeing rapidly rising numbers of cases—many related to travel, especially to France. That province's March break had started the week before, and now, as families were returning, their case numbers were soaring. The province had decided to announce restrictions on gatherings and to impose mandatory self-isolation for fourteen days on anyone returning from outside of Canada. Ontario, which was in the same boat as B.C. with respect to March break, wasn't looking to impose restrictions on returning travellers but was considering limiting mass gatherings. Across the country, all public health leaders were thinking alike on that issue after seeing how COVID-19 could spread rapidly at curling bonspiels, conferences, and so on: we agreed that restricting numbers to 250 was a reasonable place to start, but that this would have to be discussed with our respective health ministers and premiers and was therefore subject to change. The issue of travel was more complicated: our borders were a federal responsibility, and so it was up to the chief public health officer and the government of Canada to enact measures under the federal Quarantine Act.

Coming off the SAC call, I reviewed where we were with the cases in B.C.: more cases from returning travellers—from everywhere but particularly Washington State; more cases related to the dental conference; the potential for thousands of families to head off on March break into an unknown risk and to bring that risk back. Things were changing rapidly around the world as countries had started imposing lockdowns in response to rising case numbers, often stranding travellers in place for what could be weeks or months.

I put another call in to my Washington State colleagues to gauge what was going on there; I knew they had a strong public health program but was increasingly concerned by their lack of access to testing. The state epidemiologist confirmed my worries: "We have community spread," she said right away. "A lot." Recent access to testing from the University of Washington had exposed what they'd been dreading: the virus had been silently spreading and was now affecting large numbers of people; hospitals were filling up and long-term care homes were being devastated. We'd been holding our own here in B.C., but there was no way we could keep up with the flood of cases from Washington on top of the dental conference outbreak and the potential spike in cases from travel during March break. I knew we needed to take action, and take it that very day.

I made my way to the health minister's office in the hours before our media brief that day, knowing this was a monumental decision and that we'd need to make it together. And if the minister agreed, we'd need to get approval from the premier as well. I ran through my thoughts and proposed actions with the minister and deputy minister, and we talked through the implications of each measure. We needed to let people know that they shouldn't travel outside Canada for March break—not to Europe, not to Asia, not to Washington State. Borders were a federal responsibility, but under the B.C. Public Health Act I had the authority to impose restrictions on people who returned to the province. And so I would require, under a Provincial Health Officer order, that anyone returning from outside Canada must self-isolate at home for fourteen days upon their return. We'd put provisions in place for essential workers so that they could still carry on their roles while isolating when not at work. And we would impose limits of 250 people at any gathering.

As I walked through all the considerations, the minister and deputy minister nodded. We were all struck by the enormity and the uncertainty of what lay ahead, but we knew it was the right decision. Premier Horgan agreed. Our briefings in the past weeks had given him the deep background he needed in order to understand both the rationale for our recommendations and their ramifications.

The briefing was another sombre one, as the implications of these new measures sank in. At the last minute I'd also ordered anyone who had attended the dental conference to immediately self-isolate, and if they had any symptoms to get tested; I knew that the six cases so far were the tip of the iceberg and that we needed everyone in this high-risk occupation to stay away from others so they wouldn't pass it on. This turned out to be prescient; in the end, eighty-seven cases of COVID-19 in B.C. alone were associated with the conference. Had we not ordered attendees to isolate, that number would undoubtedly have been much higher.

———

I WALKED HOME THAT evening feeling exhausted and slightly stunned. I'd been involved with research, planning, and reviewing the measures for controlling pandemics for almost thirty years, but until today I hadn't truly believed that I would ever, ever use them. And as this pandemic—officially and finally declared as such on March 11, just the day before—progressed, I also knew it wouldn't end there.

I poured myself a glass of wine and sat on my couch in silence. My sister was arriving later that night from Toronto; it would be a very different visit from the one we'd planned.

IN LYNN HENRY'S WORDS

On March 12, 2020—a Thursday almost like any other, but not quite: a Thursday that followed the Wednesday when the world named a pandemic—I happened to be flying from Toronto to Victoria for a long-anticipated visit with my sister Bonnie. I wasn't the only one making the trek: our sixteen-year-old niece, Ella, and seventeen-year-old nephew, David, would arrive the day after me, flying across the country from their home on Prince Edward Island, along with their mother, our younger sister Sarah. Our grand idea, a year in the hatching, was to spend March break together, introducing the teenagers to the West Coast while subjecting them to some "quality time" with their aunts.

I had worked a full day in the offices of my publishing house and boarded an evening flight direct to Victoria. I was tired and distracted, having just finalized a major, lengthy, and convoluted book deal while sending two manuscripts to typesetting, and not for the first time that week wondered if I should be travelling at all. This was a question I had asked my sister—surely in the know; no, more than that: surely one of our country's architects of whatever plan there might be to get us through a pandemic—several times by text and phone: "Are you certain we should still do this?" The answer, invariably, perhaps impatiently: "Yes, yes. Come."

In the days to follow she would tell me, simply, "I needed family." Half rueful explanation, half gentle lament.

It wasn't until three weeks later that I would learn from her loquacious upstairs tenant, during a casual chat (from a rigorously safe distance) on a sunny morning while standing under a faintly blushing cloud of cherry blossoms, that in the days before I arrived an anonymous man had been calling Bonnie at home and threatening her. When he recited her address and declared he would show up at her door, she had reluctantly asked for protection. The next night, her tenant had answered a knock to find the police patrolling the front porch. My sister had not told me any of this when I arrived, and when I asked her about it, she gave a small shrug. "It's okay. We handled it. People are worried. They act out."

At the Toronto airport that Thursday, there were far fewer people than usual going through security; the guards had an air of jokey boredom (with each other) combined with a wary vigilance (of everyone else). In the waiting hall, people scrupulously wheeled their luggage in swooping arcs away from others. The plane itself was perhaps half full, and for once, hallelujah, there remained an empty middle seat between me at the window and my row mate on the aisle—a young woman who quickly fished out of her bag a bottle of Purell and wiped down her headrest, armrests, and tray. She kindly offered me a sanitized Handi Wipe to do the same and smiled before pulling on a cloth mask, plugging in earphones, and flipping open a magazine. It dawned on me only as the plane took off that almost every row had an empty middle seat.

Flying across the night sky, stubbornly awake in the hushed and dimmed cabin, periodically and perfunctorily offered small bottles of water ("to wash your hands if you like") by the masked and gloved, I had the eerie feeling that I was passing not through a scarf of air above the earth, gazing down to read our planet's long story of upheavals in its plains and glaciers, its mountains and inland seas, but from one dimension of time into another, a dimension with a different, slowing beat, so that all objects and subjects remained familiar, all the world's things and beings, but their importance and relevance and significance and perspective had suddenly, radically shifted.

IT WAS NEAR MIDNIGHT in B.C. when the taxi pulled up to my sister's house in a seaside neighbourhood of Victoria. During the half-hour ride from the airport, as the car whisked along the empty highway and soundlessly into town—past my sister's office building on Blanshard where it glanced sideways at Chinatown, past the gingerbread-house lights icing the legislature and a spatter of stars reflecting in the harbour, past the weathered family of totem poles still talking to land and sky beside the shut-down, concrete-clad museum—I had scrolled through a string of urgent emails from downtown Toronto. Our office building was to close. Most of us would work remotely, from home, for the indefinite future. I reached inside my hand luggage to touch the reassuring cold metal of my laptop.

The porch light flicked on and Bonnie stepped out to hug me. She was wearing light cotton sweats and holding a half glass of white wine, and her face had an odd expression. I think now that it was part heartsick shock, part self-deprecating bemusement, part utter disbelief. That afternoon, at her daily televised press conference, she'd taken the bold, controversial, potentially unpopular step of restricting travel, asking the people of British Columbia not to leave Canada for March break—only three days before that much-anticipated holiday was to begin. In part, this decision arose out of a piece of great luck for B.C.: the province's March break was happening two weeks later than a similar break in Quebec—and alarming news of infection among returning travellers, especially those coming home from trips to France and greater Europe, was being shared among senior public health officers nationally.

"I've trained for this moment for a good part of my life," Bonnie would tell me a few days later. I was following her around the kitchen and living room, trying not to annoy her while asking questions and scribbling her answers in a notebook. Days before my trip, I had been asked by a publisher back in Toronto to extract from my sister a new introduction to a book she'd written a decade earlier on public health, a book that was now being re-released. The process of word-pulling was proving trickier than I had anticipated (I'd quickly realized there was no chance of Bonnie sitting calmly at her computer, dashing off lines of crisp copy), and I had decided the only solution was to catch her thoughts on the fly and pin them to the page myself. "I've attended conferences around the world, I've consulted and planned and consulted again. I've helped write up pandemic protocols." She stopped and looked at me, then nodded quizzically at my notebook. Actually, as I was suddenly, guiltily aware, *her* notebook: a soft sky-blue one debossed with the words *Alice's Adventures in Wonderland* that I had found in a cabinet beside the kitchen table. She sighed. "But I never, ever, *ever* thought I would put them into action like this."

On the night I arrived, though, she said nothing like this. Instead, she ushered me in, waved me and my luggage towards her den-turned-spare-room, and poured me a matching small glass of wine, a nightcap. Then she curled up wearily on her favourite spot in the living room, a silvery velvet chaise longue.

I raised my glass to her and smiled. "Our mother says you look tired."

Bonnie grimaced. "I wish people would stop telling me that."

BACK IN PRINCE EDWARD ISLAND, where our parents live in Charlottetown, our ever-supportive mother, Susan, had for weeks been watching Bonnie's press conferences online. "She's amazing at answering questions," my mother had told me, her voice a mix of wonder, pride, and slight uncertainty (an emotion inevitably attached, in our family, to any public display or accomplishment), during one of my regular Sunday calls with my parents.

Bonnie had begun insisting on holding these press briefings—weekly affairs at first, almost daily by now—at the end of January. One evening halfway through my visit, she described the series of events that had led to that first briefing back on January 23. It was late March by then, and she and I were sitting at her kitchen table as the slim margin of the day's remaining sun serenely transited the window opposite us. She had just finished the last of her now daily phone conferences (this one with her local colleagues, the regional B.C. public health officers, a call she usually took at home before supper) and had removed her earbuds with a sigh, set her laptop on the bench beside the table, and poured herself a glass of very good white wine. I could faintly hear her neighbours on their shockingly (to my winter-muted Toronto eyes) verdant springtime porches, vigorously banging steel pots and brass bowls with spoons and sticks in a tinny shared rhythm, as they did every night now in support of healthcare and essential workers. Often we would step outside and join in, but this time Bonnie did not shift in her spot. She took a sip of wine, then spoke.

"In January," she said, "many people were thinking this outbreak would be confined to Wuhan in China. But I started talking to Minister Dix about what we should do when it spread. *When*, not if."

As Bonnie told me her story, the shadow of something long-forgotten took shape in my mind. It was a memory of the only other time I had directly witnessed her public health work. In June 2003, at the midpoint of the SARS epidemic, I was visiting Bonnie in Toronto from my then home in Vancouver, staying at her apartment for a couple of nights while I attended a conference. But I barely glimpsed her, and when I did she was exhausted and distracted, only just able to cook a meal, as she so loved to do, tend the containers of herbs she was growing that hot summer, read a little, sleep a little less. She also didn't say much about her work; part of the reason for that, I am certain, was confidentiality and security (later I learned that, among her other responsibilities, she had overseen the care and contact tracing for the initial cluster of cases around a traveller who had returned from Hong Kong). But I also had the sense that the effort of talking about the crisis might have caused her mental and emotional scaffolding to buckle and collapse, even as tough-minded as I knew her to be. On my final day, she invited me to join her for a quick goodbye lunch. I was to meet her on the eleventh floor of the public health building downtown, where she was leading the city's operational response to SARS under the direction of the extraordinary, empathetic, and impressive (and today much missed) Dr. Sheela Basrur, who became one of the acknowledged heroes of that epidemic.

Now, almost two decades later, as I listened to my sister describe the events and decisions that had led to B.C.'s first coronavirus press conference, I saw in my mind's eye one particular scene from that mid-SARS Toronto visit: Bonnie leading me through a warren of cubicles and offices into a quiet, windowless boardroom, where we paused for a few minutes while she consulted urgently with colleagues. Left on my own, my eye was drawn to the far wall, which featured a whiteboard bristling from end to end with Post-it Notes of various colours, connected by thin, unbroken lines of black ink. As I stared at this strangely beautiful abstraction, its meaning slowly came into focus: this was the track of the terrible disease itself, and these colours were the stages of its relentless progress within the web of people it had infected.

At the kitchen table in Victoria, half an ear tuned to my sister's voice, I was haunted by the memory of the rainbow of notes on that whiteboard, its eerie combination of the precise and mathematical with the fragile and individual. It occurred to me that now, in March 2020, the entire globe existed somewhere as yet undiscovered on that chart—in the twilight space between those poles of the coolly abstract and the shockingly personal. And that we were dependent upon the few—like Bonnie, quite possibly; like others with clear, steady voices that were beginning to sound—who could effectively articulate and traverse that space for us, with us, and hopefully one small step ahead of us.

"And so," Bonnie was saying, "I downloaded a video recording of another press briefing, one that had just happened elsewhere, and I said to Minister Dix, 'I think this should be exactly how we *not* do it.'"

"Right," I said quickly. "Of course. So, you *didn't* do it . . . how, exactly?"

Bonnie glanced at me, then patiently backtracked. "Well, like I said, we discussed that in our first press conference we should set the precedent and procedure for how we wanted to do things going forward. Because what I knew even back in January was that we would indeed be going forward, maybe only for weeks, but who knows, maybe months. And consistency of communication—not only what we said, but how and where and when and how often and regularly we said it—would be important. So, I suggested we should not have too many speakers, and not have different speakers all the time, and not be sitting behind a table. Instead, we would stand. And there would be only the two of us as the front-people, that's all. And we'd coordinate our specific message for that day, and take turns delivering it, one of us going up to the podium, then the other. The minister would always begin with acknowledgments of the land and the people we serve, and then would introduce me. I would always address the public health issues and directives—and hopefully, by the way we stood in proximity to each other, people would know that these were supported by the minister—and he would address policy and politics and especially any financial and budgetary concerns. We'd speak altogether for maybe fifteen or twenty minutes. And then we would take questions jointly."

I nodded. This description fit the choreography of the press conferences I had seen over the past couple of weeks. I, like so many others (judging from comments online and in newspaper articles about the briefings, and often about Bonnie specifically, that were now being written with alarming frequency), found the media updates oddly soothing despite their tremendously distressing content. People tended to attribute this to Bonnie's straightforward, even gripping delivery (because one sensed, rightly, that she herself was deeply interested and invested) of the facts and the science, and her articulate, calming voice. I suspected it also had to do with pure storytelling instinct: Bonnie and Minister Dix had carefully crafted a basic structure that worked, and could be repeated like a picture book, so that one knew what to expect and exactly where the surprises, even jarring ones, might be sprung on you. The hardest piece, I thought, was potentially the Q&A, but as my mother had foretold, Bonnie frankly astonished me day after day with her fluency. She would actually *listen* to a question, and then (even more impressive) actually answer it, rarely caught by surprise, often lighting up and keenly introducing a chorus of supporting detail, as if secretly happy the issue had been raised at last (the result, I knew, of a truly nerdy interest in the science and data, but also, crucially, a longtime, close working relationship with the similarly invested, committed, and passionate scientists at the B.C. Centre for Disease Control).

"That first time *was* difficult, though," Bonnie added wistfully, and I saw a flicker of her old worry from New Year's Eve, a time that now seemed impossible to conjure, like a dream just before waking. "I began by working with the deputy minister just to raise the idea that this virus needed to be paid attention to, was serious, could affect everything and everyone in this province—maybe even before the rest of the country because of our proximity to Asia, our different kinds of potentially at-risk populations who travel. To his credit, Minister Dix heard me and the deputy out, and he brought the issue forward to the premier, and they both agreed to the media briefing. But the minister was still, quite rightly, full of questions about the way we'd set it up—he wasn't entirely sure, at first, about who should speak about the public health and science part of the message. I figure this is because we'd been a bit out of step over our overdose crisis communication, and we hadn't worked together long enough to build the trust between us that there is now."

Again, a flash of memory: a couple of years ago, in Lisbon, Portugal, Bonnie in the late-afternoon July sun as we sat in a narrow funicular climbing a steep stone incline in the centre of that city. We were on our way to join others for the traditional beer and snack before a siesta and late dinner. In recent years she had often invited me to tag along with a little group of close friends with whom she liked to travel, when work allowed. As we slowly ascended past twisting streets, she told me about Portugal's progressive experiment in decriminalizing the possession of small amounts of otherwise illegal drugs. This was the first I'd heard of the approach—and so, much in the way she would later answer COVID-19 questions at press briefings, she launched rather enthusiastically into an explanation of the trial and its fascinating results so far, explaining why many of the positive outcomes weren't as counterintuitive as they might seem.

Now Bonnie frowned for a second. "But then I stepped towards that podium the minister and I had agreed on, and I spoke about what I know, and about what we didn't know yet, and about what we could do and should do and might need to do—and it was like he relaxed and said, 'Aha!'" She gave me a puckish half smile. "And now, as you know, we're a team in this."

I raised my glass, and Bonnie tilted hers towards me and got up to find a pot—not for dinner quite yet, alas, but to briefly join the lingering essential-worker supporters from the safety of her back stoop (a man with a trumpet had shown up, extending the moment into a hippie-ish, physically distant street jam) before the last of the sun disappeared.

THE NIGHT OF MARCH 12, when I arrived in Victoria and considered the state of my sister as she collapsed on her chaise longue, I knew nothing yet of what had led up to that first press conference. I had seen only a single clip from a briefing of hers—and that one only because it had become unavoidable in the previous week if you paid any attention to the national news: it captured a moment of emotion over the tragedy that was building in long-term care homes, a moment that had unexpectedly fluttered up and become trapped in a sticky loop of camera time, repeated and rebroadcast and requoted, with Bonnie's voice—both her halting words and her silence as she restrained tears—echoing round and round until it reached even my radio in Toronto as I got up for work one morning. I remember stopping cold on my way to the shower. What was this? It was strange enough that I had become used to hearing my sister's voice as background noise, often drifting into my ear from a news story as I surfaced from sleep. Now this particular, devastating clip had turned Bonnie into a symbol of the pandemic's emotional toll—precisely the kind of symbol, I knew, that she most fervently would not want to be, even if people saw it as the expression of empathy for elderly people and their caregivers that it truly was. For a few days it seemed that on every screen, there she was, tearing up, struggling to speak, and my heart would judder to a halt, waiting for her to regain composure and the flow of regular life to resume.

Looking at Bonnie in person now, watching as she moved aside a cushion and got up after a few distracted minutes of chatter about family and went to her room to consider what to wear for the next day's series of meetings and briefings, apologetically explaining that she would be up for her first phone call at five a.m. (one with public health officers from all the provinces, where the three-hour time difference between B.C. and the centre of the country did not work in her favour) and would crash at any moment and so must say goodnight, I understood for the first time that in the jump cut between that tearing-up moment and tonight, nothing regular about life had, or maybe ever would be, resumed. The new world that had slipped into focus during her tears and choked silence was precisely the one we were living in now, not the familiar old world briefly conjured back by the careful quips to reporters that followed. And the person who ducked her head back around the bedroom door to ask my opinion about this colourful blouse over that one was, in fact, walking through wilderness, emotionally drained but determined, with no choice that she could see except to keep putting one foot in front of the other, just as she had done for weeks by then. ("Do you know, this is my sixty-eighth day of work without a break?" she had said casually, as if embarrassed but compelled to mention it, as she was leaving the living room.) Now Bonnie was waving two pairs of shoes at me, one in each hand, and giving me a quizzical look. Wearing kick-ass shoes, it seemed, helped her keep moving.

(A while later, I happened upon a wide range of online responses to Bonnie's tearing-up moment. It was as if I were reading about a person I barely knew, a figure upon whom many had projected their own thoughts and fears. One comment that stayed with me was *Clearly she knows something we don't*. This struck me as not quite right, but it wasn't wrong, either. The implication was that Bonnie was deliberately withholding facts—and that, I knew, was simply not true. At the same time, she really *did* know something that others might not. She knew it from her scarring experience with SARS, from her time in Uganda helping to manage an outbreak of Ebola. What the camera had captured, and what others instinctively, perhaps subconsciously, understood they were witnessing, was the precise moment Bonnie knew we were in it for good, that there was no way back from the precipice, that a still-unknown number of people, and often those with the fewest societal and economic supports, would fall ill, that some of our most vulnerable—increasingly, it was becoming clear, older people, whom Bonnie deliberately addressed as "our elders" in acknowledgment of their value and the collective tragedy of this loss— would die, even as their families and their caregivers also suffered. The possibility long imagined, studied, and anticipated, but still never completely believed, had come to pass.)

"Oh, one more thing," Bonnie said before closing her bedroom door. "I need to leave for Vancouver and my Friday meeting with the minister right after my calls in the morning. I'm sorry, but I'll be away tomorrow night, too, and won't be getting back until Saturday after our noon press briefing. So you'll have to go by yourself to meet Sarah and the kids tomorrow when they get in from PEI, and take them to their hotel."

I silently wondered, for the final time that long day, about the wisdom of following through on our grand tour and flying our niece and nephew across the country—especially mere hours after Bonnie herself had put out-of-country travel restrictions in place for her province. But I said nothing; the last thing my sister needed was another problem or contradiction pointed out to her, one she was no doubt aware of. And who knew, perhaps she'd find comfort in having us all together over the next uncertain week. (In retrospect, when considering the confusion of this time and the struggle to decide what to do, I think of an offhand comment Bonnie made to me about some other seeming contradiction, now long forgotten. It's her words that stuck: "There's science, and there's emotion. The scientific facts are one thing; the social choices and consequences are another. We need to consider both.")

I nodded and went to the kitchen to get a glass of water and marvel at the cherry tree in bloom outside in the moonlight; booted up my laptop and sat briefly in its glow, just to check that all was okay back at my shut-down workplace in Toronto; then closed the machine's silver shell and went to bed, too, not yet knowing that within days every carefully made plan would tumble into the widening gap of the slowing-down world, and that this would become my nightly routine for weeks to come.

THE NEXT MORNING, I stumbled out of the spare room around seven, hearing the murmur of Bonnie's voice in the kitchen. She placed her finger to her lips to signal that she was on a call and pointed to the coffee maker. As I poured a cup, she put the call on speakerphone. A man's voice: pleasant, confident, and respectful, with a slight accent. I listened as he and Bonnie talked quickly, exchanging detailed health information in a kind of shorthand clearly familiar to them both; it was the conversation of two people who understood each other.

"The deputy minister," Bonnie explained when the call

ended efficiently a few minutes later. She glanced at her watch. "And I need to leave for Vancouver in twenty minutes." She sighed. "One more call, and then there's something I have to tell you." She dialed a number, and this time I could hear only her side of the conversation as she consoled someone in her carefully modulated low tone, the one she used to signal calm, saying it would all be fine; the important thing was to isolate. "So that was my executive assistant," she said with resignation when the call ended. "She just returned from a cruise, and she's all right, but someone else on the boat tested positive. I told her she has to stay home for two weeks and not be in contact with anyone. She feels bad, and yes, the timing is terrible, but what can you do. I'll miss her, though." She gathered up her cream-and-pink tartan coat and her computer and small overnight bag and stepped out the kitchen's back door. It was still inky dark outside, but an arc of lighter blue was washing across the top of the sky near a pale half-eaten wafer of moon. She was headed to the Helijet terminal a brisk ten-minute walk away along Dallas Road. Bonnie has suffered since childhood from motion sickness (a truly terrible affliction for her to have, since as children we'd moved around the country often, usually by car, when we changed homes every two years or so; and then later she had chosen to go through medical school with the navy, spending time aboard ship in all kinds of weather), and travelling by helicopter was easier on her than the other option, a harbour float plane.

Partway down the walkway she turned, remembering what she'd meant to tell me. "I know it's disappointing, but I cancelled our tickets to Vancouver and to the hockey game. The kids will just have to stay here in Victoria for the visit. There can't be any more going back and forth, I'm afraid. Unless it's absolutely necessary. I don't even know how much longer the minister and I can do it." She gave me a wave and was gone.

As it transpired, cancelling a trip across the water to Vancouver was the least of the changes to follow. By Saturday, March 14, when my sister Sarah and my niece and nephew, newly arrived, strolled in our little family bubble along the seawall and down to the Helijet terminal in the late-afternoon sunshine to welcome Bonnie back, the virus had yet again radically mutated scientists' understanding of the air we breathe.

On Sunday morning, when I got up in the semi-darkness— a line of bright red cracking open above the cherry tree outside the window—Bonnie was already in her spot at the kitchen table, tapping on her laptop. "Oh dear," she said.

"Oh dear what?"

"Oh dear, what's happening in the States." She frowned. "I hope all the snowbirds don't come home at once." She got up to make more coffee, and as it brewed she said baldly, in a rare admission of her mental state, "I'm anxious today." Then: "I think we should send Sarah and the kids home."

"Really? They've only been here two days . . ."

"Yes," she said sadly, but with a small slip of relief. "I'm going to change their tickets now."

Later I would come to understand what Bonnie couldn't tell me outright that morning: in Vancouver the day before, she and the health minister and his team had discussed closing international border points to non-Canadians and restricting flights, even as a parallel discussion was happening within the offices of the federal government. Now on Sunday, March 15, as I accompanied Sarah and my niece and nephew to Mile Zero, the westernmost point in Canada, and took photos of them beside the statue of Terry Fox forever in mid-stride there, to be posted later on social media (my nephew frowning and gazing resolutely to the side, my niece posing with hand on hip and smiling brightly at the camera in cheeky contrast), Bonnie was on the phone with her national counterparts, finalizing the details of the travel ban announcement that would be made the next day. And as the teenagers and I picked our way along the narrow, brambly path above the seawall, smiling and stepping conscientiously away from other walkers, towards a tall, slim totem pole—older than twice the combined ages of my niece and nephew, a wood-carved encyclopedia of weather—that gazes out towards the Olympic Mountains on the Washington side of the Strait of Juan de Fuca, Bonnie was absorbing with shock and distress the disastrous implications of an international dentists' conference in Vancouver that had somehow snuck past her notice as well as that of her network of colleagues in public health.

That evening over dinner in a tucked-away family booth at a favourite neighbourhood bistro—although none of us knew it then, it would be our second-last meal in a public place for months—Bonnie was close to despair. "I shouldn't have said what I did about Whistler in the briefing yesterday," she told us. In an attempt to encourage people to maintain physical distance but continue going outdoors for exercise and their mental health, she had mentioned the value of taking walks in the province's parks and enjoying the famous ski hills. Almost immediately, the operators of those hills had shut down their resorts and lifts.

"Ugh," I sympathized. "Well, I do get why they're right to do that. But your larger point is correct, too. That's the important message, don't you think?" But Bonnie was inconsolably annoyed with herself; she understood how closely every word she uttered was scrutinized. Moreover, she knew that words mattered more than almost anything else right now—that in this moment, word and action stood right beside each other. And for Bonnie, this wasn't just a hunch or instinct or vague theory. It was long-studied, deeply held gospel, informed by her experiences in fighting community transmission of deadly disease—not only SARS but also Ebola, where an ill-considered word could lead to vulnerable people being shunned, and by extension, like ripples on the surface after a rock is tossed into a pond, a widening part of the population endangered. More subtly but importantly, it was a conviction that had been formed by a lifetime of reading widely. This particular moment was only a premonitory glimpse, but I would have ample occasion over the following weeks to witness and think more about the precise influence of that reading on Bonnie's and the ministry's rhetoric.

That night, however, enough had been said; perhaps too much had been said. After dinner we strolled home in sober silence through the quieter and quieter streets.

THE EARLIEST RETURN FLIGHTS to PEI that Bonnie had been able to wrangle for Sarah and the teenagers were for Wednesday morning. Although they were disappointed to go home early, my family accepted the news with grace and even a touch of relief. Already a prickling worry had crept in: Bonnie had carefully, with studied calm, revealed to us that our tiny home province of Prince Edward Island had recorded its first case of the virus, and although our parents were in no imminent danger, even this little flare felt like a sign: go home, go home, while you still can.

We made plans to have a goodbye meal together at a popular downtown restaurant on Monday evening. Over the intervening day the city slowed and shuttered, its facade adjusting just enough for the change to be perceptible hour by hour, as if its secret inner life, with its whorl of repeating patterns and customs (horse-drawn buggies circling a postcard path for tourists; three generations bounding, walking, huffing up the front steps of the Empress Hotel for tea; a seniors' group striding purposefully through groupings of geese and flowers in Beacon Hill Park; sun-seared buskers in knee-less jeans placing upside-down hats to collect change in the inner harbour; running shoes passing baby strollers passing silicone-wheeled walkers along the widest part of windy, wave-watching Dallas Road; night wanderers weaving past a huddle of people sleeping in doorways clustered along the shade edge of the harbour wall; men in suits and women suitably dressed—like my sister right there, waiting for the light to change on the other side of the street from the long stretch of legislature lawn, having walked the ten minutes from her office through the centre of town on her way to meet the minister and plan the day's briefing), had become the subject of a time-lapse film capturing the final brief and vanishing phase of its existence. While Bonnie was at work, I walked with my sister and niece and nephew past the harbour towards Chinatown, passing regular groups of people sitting, talking, lounging, strumming—all observing appropriate distances from each other—on and between long wooden benches; a few hours later, repeating the same steps in the other direction, only one older man, perched on the edge of a stone half-wall and smoking a pungent joint, and a young couple, laughing quietly at their phones on either side of a manicured planter, remained on that usually crowded mall.

Perhaps this was why, on Monday night, it was shocking to discover that the restaurant where we'd reserved a spot was packed with patrons—as if we'd stumbled into a surprise underground party after believing everyone had long gone home. Signs on the door sternly asked people to reserve ahead, stay away if sick, and observe physical distancing rules, but once that door opened, a burst of music and laughter rushed out into the spring evening. Indeed, the place seemed unchanged from my last visit years ago: pleasantly dim and warm, crammed and bustling. As Sarah, the teenagers, and I followed our server to a table tucked into an alcove, we couldn't help brushing the backs of chairs and people as we passed. Bonnie was to join us halfway through the meal, after finishing some last calls at her office, and I felt suddenly worried. People had begun to recognize her face on the street, and what if she was seen and called out for being in a venue that didn't— couldn't possibly, with its current set-up—practise the rules she'd been pleading for all to observe? And most concerningly, surely this was dangerous for us, for everybody?

I watched the server dance towards us, twisting her body between tables, tray of food held high, just as Bonnie appeared and quietly drew up a chair. She situated herself at the end of the table facing in towards us and the alcove, the back of her head towards the open room. She said nothing about the tables and diners pressed up against each other in the centre of the room, and we chatted about our own small adventures and worries that day—the last few purchases the teenagers had made, sometimes minutes before a store was closing up for the foreseeable future; the anticipated strangeness and worry of the flight home. But after Bonnie and I had hugged our soon-to-be PEI-bound family, who were staying at a hotel nearby, and were strolling back to her house, she winced and said, "I've resisted doing this, but I guess I may have to order restaurants to close. It simply isn't possible to keep people apart in that atmosphere, is it?"

I could hear the hesitation and regret—and understood this to be both a professional and personal dilemma, for there could be few more ardent supporters of good food and fine company than my sister. But I nodded. As we crossed the silent street—now, like all roads in this point of land between the dark silhouette of the park and the restless sea, absent of cars and people at night—and entered Bonnie's home, I thought how the world had so quickly shrunk to this: this porch, these rooms, this person. And how fortunate I was with just this: my welcoming porch, my lighted rooms, my human connection.

"I've been thinking," I said.

"Me, too," said Bonnie briskly. "I've been thinking you should go spend this time with our parents. Everyone safe in one place. Get out to PEI while you still can."

"Ah," I said. "Hmm. Well, I've been thinking I should stay here with you for a while longer than we planned, instead of returning to Toronto right away. To support you, if I can. I have my computer and manuscripts and access to everything I need for work. And I have an idea . . . I just think it might be good for you to have someone here, to witness and know what you're doing. And our parents will be relieved we're together. For a few weeks, anyhow."

Bonnie frowned and turned to look out the living-room window at the darkening homes across the way. She pulled on the cord of the blind so that only a small deep-blue rectangle of sky at the top of the windowpane remained visible. The stoic face of a rising moon gazed in on us, unreadable, and I remembered that what we see of that orb from here on Earth, its news of the universe travelling through space, is always a slight stutter in the past. The moon, one breath ahead of us. What did it know now?

"Okay," my sister said. "Yes." She turned back to the glow of the room. "Stay." Then she held up two fingers in the shape of a *V* and gave me a wry half smile. "But you have to understand: I won't be thinking about anything except COVID-19. Imagine my forehead tattooed with a big *V* for virus. That's my whole life now."

PART II

BE CALM

{ Week Two: Before and After March 17 }

IN DR. BONNIE HENRY'S WORDS

F riday, March 13: after saying a quick hello and goodbye to my sister Lynn, newly arrived at my home in Victoria, I flew to Vancouver for the day's meetings and media brief, which as usual was to be held jointly with B.C.'s health minister.

As I got off the flight and was walking through the terminal, my eye caught the television headlines: our prime minister's wife had become ill and tested positive for COVID-19 after an exposure at an event in London, England. It represented another confirmation that the virus was everywhere, even in high places; several others at the event had also become ill. Now Sophie Grégoire Trudeau was in isolation at home in Ottawa, with Trudeau himself in quarantine in a separate area of their house. Almost immediately he began holding daily briefings from a temporary podium in a tent outside their door. Seemingly overnight, this virus had become very real for all Canadians. And its relentless spread to countries once thought impenetrable, and to people thought to somehow be above risk, continued.

In the days following my orders on March 12—orders that restricted gatherings and required anyone returning to British

Columbia to self-isolate for fourteen days, along with strong advice not to travel at all—time seemed to slow to a crawl. The orders' implications were sinking in across all sectors of our community, particularly those families who'd planned to travel for March break. But I knew these measures were only the beginning. We now needed to prepare in earnest: cases were rapidly rising, and what was unfolding in places like Northern Italy and even closer in New York City—where the same story we had seen in Italy was repeating itself, hospitals filling up, ambulances being turned away from emergency entrances, provisions made for field hospitals in Central Park and mass graves on Riker's Island—was an all too real possibility for Canada.

On that morning's flight to Vancouver I was still feeling slightly numb from the magnitude of what I'd just put into place, even while realizing that there would need to be further restrictions to come. As new outbreaks were being detected, my colleagues and I were seeing more unlinked community cases and more tragic deaths in our long-term care homes. In thinking over the decisions of the day before, I knew in my heart we were on the necessary path. Yet I also knew that my internal bias is to minimize risks and to be overly optimistic, so over the previous few days I'd also checked in regularly with wise people: my medical health officer colleagues on the front lines, the deputy minister, my mentor and predecessor Dr. Kendall, and my contacts at the WHO and in the U.S. and U.K. We didn't always agree, but the discussion and debate always gave me more insight into the issues and into the underpinnings of my own response.

During those endless days of early March, thoughts of what was happening, of what we needed to do, of what I could not yet see about this virus silently moving through our communities swirled in my mind constantly and made sleep an unattainable dream. From my experience in previous crises, I was well aware that we in public health would inevitably be accused, on the one hand, of not doing enough and, on the other hand, of over-reacting. This wasn't my first pandemic—and while my aim was to impose only the restrictions needed to manage the virus, and no more than that, I also knew that the "perfect" response was never possible.

After the SARS outbreak in 2003, I'd spent many, many hours on developing and understanding public health ethics— the explicit moral underpinnings of the decisions we made. Now the overriding principle resonating in my thoughts was that of "least restrictive means": doing just what was needed, and only what was necessary, to prevent illness and death. But with all we were learning about this new virus—its transmission, its death rates, and the course of its illness—I realized that we had to be on the side of seemingly overreacting. After all, the devastating impact of not doing enough, early enough, was playing out in more and more cities and countries around the world. And I knew that when the healthcare system was overwhelmed, people died—and not just from COVID-19, but because they couldn't get the medical care they needed for the myriad other health issues that continued to affect them. When that happened, the economy was also threatened. Sick people can't work, and if essential services were disrupted, the cost in lives would only escalate. In the end, economies could be resuscitated. But lives, once taken, would never come back. I knew there would be negative consequences to any decision we made, and inevitably there'd be suffering, whether from COVID-19 itself or from lack of access to healthcare or from the shuttering of businesses and schools, and the uncertainty and

economic devastation this would cause. It was a haunting realization for me—whatever we did would cause harm—and it
was impossible to know in this moment exactly what would
cause the least harm.

On that morning of Friday the 13th, the news, and my
email, were full of inevitable, understandable pushback and
general disbelief at the restrictions we'd announced the day
before—particularly from the cruise lines and air travel industry, who could foresee devastation for their businesses. Just as
I'd expected, I was accused of overreacting. But I knew that
soon, as a wave of returning travellers became ill across the
country, the risk would become clear.

Very quickly I also realized that if we continued to test
everyone who came home with respiratory symptoms, our limited testing capacity would be overwhelmed. We were still in
influenza season, seeing lots of flu as well as other respiratory
viruses. (Indeed, in the end, for every hundred tests done in
March and into April, twenty would be positive for influenza
and only one, on average, would be positive for COVID-19.) In
early March I'd already begun considering that we'd need to
focus our testing on where it was needed most. This was
becoming clear at a time, however, when the WHO, on the
other hand, was admonishing countries to "test, test, test!"

By March 14, watching the devastation happening in Italy
and in New York City as people with COVID flooded hospitals and intensive care units, I understood that our singular focus
needed to become the protection of the healthcare system—and
this meant adapting our testing strategy so that those who most
needed a test could get one as quickly as possible. In the week
to follow, we in B.C. public health would shift from testing
anyone with symptoms to testing only those who were likely to

need hospital care, who were healthcare workers, or who were in long-term care. While we knew there were inevitably going to be returning travellers with COVID-19, the order I had issued meant that all these people were already required to isolate when they returned so that, if they did become sick, they wouldn't pass the virus on to others. That was the most important consideration in gaining some control over this rapidly growing outbreak, and one of the key reasons I had issued my March 12 order.

Over the next days we would also learn that most people with the virus had very mild illness, especially the young and healthy, and could be safely managed at home. And so we ramped up our nurse line, one that people across the province could call for consultation and triage. Only those who were showing symptoms that might need hospital care would be sent for a test. While this would clearly lead to an underestimation of how much COVID-19 illness there was in our communities, we had to balance that against making sure that those who needed a test could get one.

This shift made perfect sense to those of us who worked in public health, as well as our teams in the lab and hospitals, but delivering the message to the public—especially given the WHO pronouncements and the race in other provinces and territories to test as many people as possible—proved challenging. Soon, day after day in the press briefings with the minister, I was asked about testing: Why were we not testing everyone? What was our testing capacity? Why were we not keeping up with the others? Why were we not following what the WHO advised?

I knew we had to hold the line on testing or risk dangerous delays helping those who most needed one. A delay could result in serious changes to the care ultimately required, whereas proper access to testing would not only ensure that the most vulnerable were treated in a timely way but that health-care workers and everyone already in our health system were also protected. Meanwhile, our public health laboratory was working flat out, seven days a week, and transferring their vital findings to labs in hospitals across the province. Slowly but surely, we were expanding our network and capacity.

Over the past week, as more and more people had tested positive, I'd made a key change in our daily media briefing. Now, instead of providing limited details on every individual case, I was reporting on aggregate numbers: the number of people who'd tested positive and where they were located in the province. I knew, of course, that reporting only those who'd tested positive would underestimate the true number of people with COVID-19 in B.C. But I also realized that the "true" numbers would have to wait. All those people who'd returned from travel or had mild disease and were recovering at home would be counted later. The full extent of the infectious wave would have to be determined when antibody tests (or "serology" tests) were available at some point in the future.

Still, focusing on the wise use of our testing capacity did not spare me from the relentless media inquisition on numbers, numbers, and more numbers. This, too, was a phenomenon I knew well. Every health crisis I'd ever been involved with had sooner or later become defined by numbers and the continual search for what further meanings they could convey. Number of tests reported, number of tests pending, number of probable versus confirmed cases, number of travellers, number of healthcare workers, numbers of investigations and outbreaks, number in hospital and in ICU, number of masks we possessed—it would take an army analyzing data all the hours of the day to satisfy the need. And so, to avoid this exhausting chase of ever-changing figures, I made the decision that we would report daily on these critical few: number of tests completed and number found positive, number of confirmed cases, number of people in hospital/ICU, and number who died. And I began to seed the idea with my colleagues that we could periodically pull together much more detailed data and present it publicly so that we all could have shared knowledge about who was being affected, where, and when. I also laid the groundwork for the idea of presenting the important work we were doing on modelling, particularly at the B.C. Centre for Disease Control, to help guide our decisions. That, however, would be a challenge for another day, since not everyone on my team yet believed that the public was ready to understand models and how they could be used.

The press briefing on March 13, in a room overlooking the Vancouver harbour, was serious and intense. We'd begun practising physical distancing at these events, but on that day the room was still full of cameras and reporters, a few of whom were wearing masks. The questions Minister Dix and I faced were probing: the journalists wanted details, specifically about how we would enforce the rules for returning travellers. I also detected an undercurrent of disbelief: Did we *really* mean to say that people shouldn't travel?

Yes, I confirmed, and I renewed my call for the federal government to do their part, too, and at the least issue a national travel advisory. These matters, along with overriding concerns about our border with Washington and another long-term care outbreak, were the issues of the day and made for a comprehensive, exhausting exchange.

Afterwards, as I walked slowly back to my hotel in the March evening darkness, Vancouver was unusually quiet and still; a sense of urgency and fear was in the air. Even the hotel, bustling and full not a week before, was oddly subdued. Only three fellow travelling souls sat at the bar as I ate my dinner while answering a never-ending string of emails.

Then, when I got back to my room to finish work, I suddenly remembered that my younger sister and her children, my niece and nephew, were to have arrived in Victoria that day, joining my sister Lynn, who had arrived from Toronto the night before. I felt a pang of guilt: I'd planned our March break together, and now everything had changed. The Canucks game we'd scored tickets to months ago had been cancelled that very day (first the NBA and then the NHL had suspended their seasons). My niece and nephew had never been to the West Coast, and Lynn and I had planned so much for them to experience, from the mountains to the Gulf Islands to a tour of the university campuses. Now I wasn't certain what we would do. I fell into bed, exhausted mentally and physically. We'd work out the visit tomorrow, I told myself, when I got back home to Victoria.

ON SATURDAYS THE MINISTER and I typically held the media briefing earlier in the day than usual, but even so, our briefing on the 14th proved to be another marathon. So many dominoes were falling as travel advisories came from the federal government, sports seasons got cancelled, and across the country people retreated to their homes. We also began to hear reports of rushes on toilet paper, hand sanitizer, and Lysol wipes. Fear and anxiety led people to act out, and that included acts of hoarding. More worrisome, verbal attacks on those who looked

Asian were becoming more common. The insidious evil of "othering" was creeping in and undermining our social cohesion.

From the beginning I'd chosen my words carefully when doing media briefings. I understood that the many things we didn't yet know about this virus were causing fear, and that our natural human inclination was to fill in the gaps ourselves, creating an "imagined" epidemic fed by our own experiences, rumours, stories, the media. I also understood that some people deal with fear by assigning blame and stigmatizing the "other"— those whom they feel are responsible. And in this pandemic it was Asian people who were being increasingly targeted. Remembering the stigma that had occurred in Toronto during SARS, and in Uganda with Ebola, made me acutely aware of the power of words and of the need to draw on our common experiences and suffering to build a sense that we were all in this together. I knew, not only from my own experiences but from data collected from crises around the world, that this would in turn build community resilience. And it would be community resilience and connectedness that would help us weather this storm.

That Saturday, during the briefing, I took pains to emphasize that it was Canadians and members of our own communities who were returning home, and that while they might indeed be bringing risk of this new virus with them, we needed to support these people, our fellow citizens, to isolate in order to best protect us all. I said all this as clearly and matter-of-factly as I could, amid ever louder cries to "keep them out." After the briefing I caught my flight home to Victoria more worried than ever.

———

SUNDAYS WERE MY DAY to regroup and catch up on data, review evidence coming out around the world, and then participate in the daily national Special Advisory Committee (SAC) call. The minister and I had decided not to do Sunday media briefings unless we needed to share something urgent with the people of B.C.; this was an attempt to develop a rhythm we could sustain into the unknowable future. So, although Sunday was by no means a day off, I found it a relief not to have to prepare for cameras and questions. Speaking to the public about important issues was, and is, a key part of my role, but it was also something I needed to summon courage for each and every time. This stemmed partly from my natural tendency towards introversion and partly from the responsibility I felt knowing that any missteps could create more fear and panic, could affect people's very lives. I also knew that as things changed my words would be brought back to me, and often not in a good way. Still, I needed to be frank and open and to build trust as the storm clouds gathered. That way, as things shifted with new developments and new knowledge, the public would, I hoped, shift along with me, trusting in our process.

Early that Sunday, after another sleepless night, I was in my office in downtown Victoria. The previous afternoon, after my hop over from Vancouver, I'd met up with my visiting family, still a little jet-lagged from their flight in from Charlottetown. We'd had a lovely dinner at my favourite local restaurant, followed by a walk along the water to see the glow of the mountains and Olympic Peninsula before turning in early to bed. As I tossed and turned that night, unable to settle the uneasiness in my mind, I came to the realization that I needed to send my East Coast sister, niece, and nephew home. Things were changing rapidly across the world and across the country. We in B.C. would be putting in more restrictions in the coming days, and I knew PEI would be doing the same. I'd need to talk to Lynn, too, and make arrangements the next day.

The data I scrolled through in my office on Sunday morning did nothing to allay my fears. We had more long-term care outbreaks in the province, and it was a challenge getting enough healthy staff to come in and care for those in need, and to access the needed PPE and infection prevention and control expertise. Our pandemic in B.C., it was becoming clear, was being driven by long-term care outbreaks—and we were learning the hard way how virulent and pernicious this virus could be in those settings. Long-term care homes in B.C., like those in most of Canada and the Western world, are a combination of public and private companies, both for-profit and not-for-profit. Having arisen from the concept of "poor hospitals" in the 1800s, many were run by religious organizations to support community members as they aged and needed more care than families could provide. But as we'd soon learn, the lack of integration into our public healthcare system would prove challenging in this pandemic—challenging, and deadly.

Early on we based our response to COVID-19 in long-term care homes on the detailed protocols we'd developed to respond to annual influenza outbreaks there—but without the benefit of such key influenza interventions as antiviral medications and vaccines. With influenza, an outbreak was defined as two or more cases over a period of one week, and residents were tested if they developed any symptoms at all. But as the COVID-19 cases and, tragically, deaths rose rapidly in the first care homes where the virus appeared, it was clear that this approach wouldn't be nearly good enough. Residents were infected and dying sometimes within hours, with very minimal symptoms: feeling more tired than usual, or not being hungry, or slight confusion, but not always the cough, fever, and aches we'd expected from experience with other respiratory diseases.

We needed to adjust our response, and fast. Outbreak teams were formed, with key experts in infection control, nursing, environmental services, and epidemiology; they were led by the regional medical officers of health. Any single case in a health-care worker or a resident was categorized as an outbreak, and we moved rapidly to implement measures to prevent its spread. These included discontinuing all visits, screening everyone daily, enhancing cleaning practices, testing affected wards—and whole facilities, if needed—and isolating any ill residents. Communal dining was suspended, as were gatherings, outings, and events; nor were nonessential services allowed, and even religious support was excluded until we had evidence that the infection could be stopped.

But despite these challenging, draconian measures, transmission remained difficult to break—and people, often our seniors and elders, were dying.

That Sunday, March 15, I learned with dismay of more deaths and more affected care homes; my front-line public health leaders were telling me that the virus was spreading in the community and that cases were hard to link. Many infected people now, including healthcare workers who'd been the index, meaning the first, cases in care home outbreaks, were linked to travel to Washington State. It was also becoming clear that healthcare workers who worked at more than one care home were transporting the virus along with them. In Canada, and in B.C., we were learning, as was the rest of the world, that this virus could spread before people showed symptoms, and that in the young and healthy, symptoms could be so mild that they may not even be recognized as such. This would prove to be our greatest challenge: How could we prevent transmission of a virus that could move between people unrecognized? This dawning realization added to our collective anxiety even as the virus spread.

The news on our national SAC call that Sunday was equally dire. Across the country we were in the same storm. What was happening globally was affecting us all, but it was playing out in different ways in different regions. We had all implemented provincial travel restrictions, and now the federal government was adding national travel advisories, too. And since we were all feeling the pinch of scarce access to personal protective equipment, we agreed we needed a coordinated purchasing plan for PPE as well as for ventilators. As cases rose exponentially, our fears of overwhelming our hospitals and intensive care units grew as well. I signalled our mounting concerns in B.C., which I knew were echoed elsewhere, about rapid, stealth transmission in care homes and the need to protect our seniors and elders along with other vulnerable populations, among them people living in shelters, correctional facilities, and communal settings. These had all been critical settings in my past experience with both the 2003 SARS and the 2009 HINI influenza pandemics, and they were proving once again to be of concern. We also talked about more broad population measures: closing businesses, schools, and daycares, and sending people home for an unknown period of time—measures we'd barely dared contemplate only weeks before. "Social distancing" entered our lexicon, soon to be replaced with the much preferred "physical distancing," to add to our core messages: clean your hands, don't touch your face, cover your cough, and stay home if you're ill.

Schools were a particular concern for all of us on the SAC call. Although in B.C. I'd put measures in place to prevent people travelling for March break, we now needed to make a decision on what would happen when the break ended in two weeks. I knew from my two decades of work on pandemic planning that closing schools had many negative consequences, and that these weren't spread evenly in the population. Children who were struggling would be impacted most, and some would never catch up; this could affect their lives forever, leading to increased risk of poverty, substance use, mental health concerns, and other long-term consequences. For other children, school is the one safe place in their lives—the place where they have access to food and to health and social supports. Teachers and staff were uniquely placed to notice whether children were in danger at home and to intervene; 40 percent of reports to Children's Aid came from schools. Children with special needs were also likely to suffer disproportionately, given that most support programs for these children are based in the school setting; closing schools would prove an added burden not only on them but on their families as well. On the other hand, we still didn't know with certainty how children were affected by COVID-19 and whether they would amplify transmission in the school setting, something we knew happened with influenza. Teachers and staff were also understandably anxious about their own safety, especially those who were older or who had underlying health issues. Crowded classrooms, failing infrastructure, lack of resources for cleaning, and poor ventilation were only some of the concerns. We concluded our call acknowledging that we needed to make a decision in the coming days about what we would do so that families and teachers could plan.

I met up with my sisters and niece and nephew late that Sunday afternoon. As we walked through the downtown streets of Victoria, the city felt eerie, its shops still open but few customers inside. Uncertainty hung in the air, as if people weren't clear what had happened and what it might mean for them. In our normally bustling local bookstore, a handful of people danced around each other—reminding me that we were all still in the early awkward phase of understanding what keeping a safe distance might mean. As we sat down for dinner that evening, I explained to my PEI-based family that our world was changing and that they needed to go home, both for their sake—given the real danger of getting stranded in B.C.—but also out of concern for my parents. They, too, lived in PEI, and we needed family to be close by for support. I tried not to show my mounting anxiety, but I could see my concern reflected back in everyone's faces.

That evening we booked flights back. The soonest available were for the Wednesday morning—so at least the teenagers had two more days to experience a bit of the West Coast and spend more time with my sister Lynn. I, on the other hand, would be far too distracted to be any company, and in any case, with my days starting early and ending late, I'd have little opportunity to see them.

MONDAY MORNING BROUGHT FRESH concerns, as case numbers climbed inexorably across the country. Washington State declared a state of emergency and implemented a statewide "stay at home" order, closing schools and businesses. Meanwhile, the extent of the testing debacle in the U.S. was becoming clearer. The Centers for Disease Control and Prevention in Atlanta, whose very raison d'être was to support America in a pandemic, had erred in a monumental way. The test developed in its lab was faulty, which had led to extreme restrictions on its use—even as cases were spreading rapidly in New York, in Seattle and throughout Washington, and now in California. Because of their lab error, the virus had spread in communities across the nation undetected and unchecked.

What were our options in B.C.? I'd been going over and over them in my mind and consulting with my trusted advisers. Although I'd already enacted orders around travel and the numbers of people permitted in mass gatherings, the process to do so was cumbersome. In our exceptional, fast-evolving circumstances I needed orders to be put in place rapidly, but the provisions for reconsideration could hold things up. As I stared at the rising curve of infection, I recognized that we'd need to be nimble—and that the one step I could take to allow this was to declare a public health emergency. Minister Dix and I had recently discussed the possibility, but that Monday I brought it up again with him and Deputy Minister Stephen Brown, who agreed to think about the implications seriously. I knew it would be difficult to do, much less implement properly, without the support of the minister and the premier. And importantly I wanted to be in sync with them, if possible, especially in a pandemic whose effects, it was becoming clear, would be far-reaching.

So far no other province had taken such a step, but I also knew we were all in discussions about doing just that—and in a few critical ways, B.C. was a bit ahead of some other provinces in seeing the effects of the pandemic. Plus, whereas in most other provinces it was the premier who needed to make the declaration, B.C.'s Public Health Act allowed me to make it unilaterally. B.C. also had an Emergency Management Act that enabled the premier or the minister of public safety to declare a more general provincial state of emergency. It was used most often to deal with things like natural disasters and had been invoked extensively in 2017 and 2018, for example, during massive wildfires that affected the province. A public health emergency, on the other hand, had been declared only once before, by my predecessor in 2016, to deal with the province's ongoing overdose crisis.

On Mondays, the minister and I held our media brief early in the day so that we'd be reporting on the cases over just two periods (the numbers from Saturday and Sunday). The tally seemed less daunting that way. I was struck by the parallels in my life now to a book that had been influential in my thinking about human responses to crises: Albert Camus's *The Plague*. In it, Camus describes how, as plague cases rose in his fictional world, authorities started reporting the numbers daily to reduce fear; the figures would seem smaller that way. When I mused on this aloud to Minister Dix, he immediately understood. He was very familiar with the novel, he told me, having read it many times in the original French while living in France years before. I was bemused to think this pandemic was exposing things we otherwise might never have known we had in common.

That day's briefing was another momentous one. Numbers were up. Plus, the measures introduced the week before were sinking in, and we were being asked to provide even greater clarity and direction about what people had to do to stay safe. I laid out in detail the obligations of returning travellers: stay at home for fourteen days; call the dedicated phone number if they developed symptoms to see if a test was needed and to receive health advice. No shopping, no visiting friends and family, no going to work, no taking transit.

I knew this could only work well if we supported people as they took the necessary actions, so I spoke about the need for communities to care for each other: that this was the time to pick up groceries for a neighbour, to check on friends and especially seniors, to bring medications and food, to walk people's dogs if they were in isolation. To help each other in this crisis. I stressed that supplies could be delivered safely if dropped off in the doorway or left on the step. Assisting another person while keeping a distance was safe. I was aware that research has shown altruism to be one of the consistent social responses to emergencies, and I hoped that by putting these ideas forward people would be encouraged to act in altruistic ways.

I also announced that we'd decided to suspend in-class-room schooling once March break was over. After a two-week extension of the break, classes would return online across the province. It would be a tremendous pivot in a short period of time. But after extensive consultation, and given what we knew and didn't yet know of the virus, all of us who'd made this deci-sion were convinced it was the most reasonable option.

And since more and more settings were being linked to viral transmission in our communities and around the world, I gave additional orders: mass gatherings would be limited to a maximum of fifty people, down from 250, and even then dis-tancing needed to be maintained and measures taken to enhance cleaning. People would have to have access to hand washing and sanitizer. Screening was required to ensure that anyone who was ill did not attend. Yet even these measures wouldn't be sufficient in some venues, so after much agonizing I ordered casinos, entertainment establishments (among them movie theatres and concert halls), and recreational facilities to close. These, I knew from the evidence we'd already analyzed, were perfect environments for the inadvertent spread of COVID-19 as people crowded together indoors, often in spaces with poor ventilation.

Similar measures had been put in place in China and elsewhere in Asia, then across Europe, then in the U.S., and now in Canada. But it still seemed very personal and strange to announce their implementation at home in B.C.

My own sense of disbelief, like that of so many others, was intense. I also had the feeling that time had slowed—even while being inundated with phone calls, emails, letters, and even faxes asking for more details and expressing anger, anxiety, fear, and sometimes thanks. People wrote saying they couldn't believe that our measures applied to them. Some accused me of ruining lives: that it would be my fault if businesses failed. That the arts, from movies to plays to the symphony, would never recover.

All of this seeped into my heart and soul and left me numb. Rationally, I knew the global nature of the pandemic meant that what happened in China affected us, what happened in Italy affected us, what happened in the U.S. affected us. I hadn't been the manufacturer of this crisis. Still, it was evident that, for people in B.C., I'd become the face of the pandemic. And past experience had shown me that when people are afraid, they react in anger, or act out of anxiety, lashing out at those who they feel are responsible or who at least represent the "decision makers." As I gradually, reluctantly accepted that I'd be the subject of a range of responses, I began to consider the idea that, if we found the right message, we could channel that frustration and anger into productive action. Rather than using the stick to make people comply—measures we'd seen in the extreme in China—I believed we could bring people along, and bring them together, by acknowledging our shared suffering and urging compassion. Maybe not everyone, I thought, but most people.

Late that Monday evening I caught up with my sisters, niece, and nephew for a goodbye dinner at a favourite restaurant in Victoria. In compliance with the recent public health orders the normally bustling, crowded space was more open than usual and tables had been pulled apart; but knowing what I knew about the dangers of transmission, the space still felt close and I worried. My family had almost finished eating when I arrived, so we took my dinner to go and walked home in the early darkness. Little did I know that this would be my last restaurant meal for many months.

TUESDAY, MARCH 17—St. Patrick's Day—was a day of realization and reckoning for many people, including me.

Once again I'd started my morning early, this time to participate in a four a.m. WHO call with colleagues from around the world. The global news wasn't in the least heartening; quite the reverse. It was becoming increasingly clear that the early exponential growth seen in some cities posed the biggest risk for everyone, and that rapid spread in communities from those with minimal or no symptoms was the biggest danger. Once hospitals became overloaded, the spillover effects to the entire population were dangerously amplified. Healthcare workers became infected because they didn't have sufficient time to use their PPE properly—or, often, were short of PPE to begin with. And everyone else couldn't get care for their health needs, resulting in increased sickness and death from all causes.

Transmission in large numbers between people with mild or no symptoms was proving to be the cause of that exponential growth. But more nuanced analysis revealed this to be situational and dependent on many factors. We still didn't know why most people spread the virus to only one or two others while sometimes a person with mild or even no recognized symptoms spread it to hundreds. Such stories were surfacing now: a wedding in Germany where the father of the bride, the only known infected person, passed on the virus to over two hundred guests, some of whom died. The public health investigation showed that he'd greeted every guest with hugs and cheek kisses. What if he'd been a regular guest rather than the father of the bride, we wondered, and hadn't greeted every person: Would the same tragedy have unfolded? And closer to home was an unfortunate and now famous event in Seattle, where fifty-two out of sixty-one people who'd participated in a two-and-a-half-hour choir practice with a person showing no symptoms became infected—despite maintaining distance from each other and using hand sanitizer. How could one pre-symptomatic person spread the virus to so many?

While we figured out these important details, keeping infected people away from others would be key. In public health we generally use one metre as a safe distance for risk of transmission of droplets (this virus's means of transmission, as suggested by the research to date), but the WHO was now increasingly recommending a distance of two metres. As well, the role of non-medical masks in preventing the expulsion of droplets was being closely studied, in a positive way. What was becoming apparent to me, having been part of such discussions for more than a decade, was that we were learning more in weeks about the transmission of respiratory viruses than we had in years. And in my mind there were clear gradations of risk with distance, time, and place: outside was safer than inside, and being inside with lots of open windows and few people was safer than being in a crowd in close quarters. The global challenge, and my own particular challenge, was how to convey that nuanced message in a way that would help people make the right decisions. There was no easy answer.

Meanwhile, at home in B.C., things were moving fast. On that Tuesday, March 17, rumours of planned St. Patrick's Day parties in Vancouver that would attract large crowds in restaurants and pubs were causing concern. As the minister and I headed to our media briefing in Victoria that afternoon, I knew that the local medical health officer in Vancouver, with the support of the City, would pass an order closing bars altogether. Other municipalities were looking to do the same—and to address those groups of people who hadn't yet absorbed or accepted the restrictions we'd ordered across the province. And in the middle of all this, the safety of restaurants, bars, retail locations, hair salons—the list went on—was being questioned by staff and patrons of these establishments alike.

Now was clearly the time for me to declare a public health emergency. Such an act would focus attention on the gravity of the situation and enable me to make the necessary orders verbally as well as in writing, and as soon as possible. The minister and premier agreed without a beat. We all understood that I needed the authority not only to take action quickly but also to compel data that would help us track the movement and impact of COVID-19 throughout our province. I was struck, too, by the equal need to give people hope—to let them know that we'd weather this storm together, and that there were things each one of us could do to help ourselves and each other.

As I scribbled my notes for the media brief, words came quickly to mind, especially the word "kindness." In the way I thought about it, kindness builds community, which in turn builds resiliency. "Calm" was another word I wrote down, thinking of all we'd heard about people's increasing anxiety and frustration; how some were responding by panic-buying essentials. Finally, I scrawled the word "safe": What did we need to do to stay safe? This was clearly a question on everyone's mind. As the minister and I—and my sister Lynn, who was to be a rare guest at the briefing—made our way through the underground passage to the press room at the legislature, these three words were floating around in my head.

That day I announced the second-ever public health emergency in B.C., and followed this with add-on orders closing in-room dining in restaurants, bars, and pubs, limiting these establishments to takeout and delivery only. The gravity of the situation was sinking in at last. And as if to make the situation even more resonant, new cases were rapidly popping up in communities across the province, many related to local dental workers who'd attended the Vancouver conference less than two weeks before. There were also new deaths, most notably and sadly in long-term care.

It had been a tough few days, I acknowledged to the assembled media, and I knew without a doubt that, given the virus's incubation period, more difficult days were in store. The people who were getting sick now had been exposed up to fourteen days earlier, and the people they themselves had exposed were now at risk. I explained that what we were seeing today reflected events of the recent past, events we couldn't alter. We couldn't get angry about what had happened, or that the virus had spread between people unknowingly. But we *could* change our future, I said, if we all took measures now to prevent the next case, the next exposure. Once someone was exposed, there was nothing we could do to prevent them from getting sick if they had the misfortune to have come in contact with a high-enough dose of COVID-19; all we could do was compassionately support these people in staying home and away from others, providing them with the care they needed.

Now that we knew the virus was here—and knew how it was spreading among those we were close to, our communities and families and loved ones—everything was up to us. From this moment forward, we all needed to do what we could to determine our fate for the next two weeks. And what we could do was clear: stay home as much as possible; keep a safe distance from others outside our household; clean our hands regularly; stay away from others, even family, if we were sick; and call ahead to our healthcare providers so that assessments could be carried out safely.

Glancing down at the words I'd scribbled on a sheet of paper, I ended that sombre media briefing with a phrase that would become a hallmark of my approach to the global pandemic we were to be embroiled in for even longer than I knew: "Now is our time to be kind, to be calm, and to be safe."

THAT EVENING WAS MY final night with my PEI-bound family; my sister Lynn would be staying on to be with me through the next few critical weeks. As we cooked up a West Coast salmon dinner in my kitchen to see the travellers off, I apologized to my niece and nephew, explaining that my mind was completely preoccupied with the pandemic. What I didn't tell them was that I was having dreams where I was a maypole and people were dancing around me, wrapping me in the ribbons of all the many, many COVID-19 issues that needed solving; the ribbons were being woven around me faster than I could keep up. But once my sister Sarah and her kids had made it home, I'd be able to feel that one ribbon, at least, had been tied off safely.

On March 18 I was up before dawn, heading back to Vancouver for the next few days. This had become my pattern: Sunday to Wednesday in Victoria and the end of the week in Vancouver, flying home Saturday afternoons after that day's briefing. It was exhausting and challenging, but it meant we could connect with the community media, which were based in Vancouver, as well as the mainstream media, which tended to have people in both Vancouver and the government hub of Victoria. The minister and I had purposely spent time with the Chinese, Vietnamese, and South Asian media, going on radio talk shows and TV shows that were widely watched in those communities. This key outreach had paid off, stimulating support for community members returning from outside the province or country and getting out my message of caring and togetherness. I wanted people to receive that message directly from us as a way to help counter any attempts to blame or to "other" particular populations.

During the almost empty early morning flight, I watched the sun rise over the beauty of the Gulf Islands, Mount Baker glowing orange in the distance. Our global community had changed dramatically in ways we couldn't have imagined even a few weeks before. In the past days I'd implemented measures that affected every single person in our province, and more were to come. But there was still beauty—and I was reminded that we still needed to breathe, to embrace what we had. I knew this would be my message that afternoon: a reminder that this wouldn't be forever, that we were in this together, that there was hope.

Behind the scenes we continued to receive reports of people panic-buying food, staples, medications, and toilet paper. What had begun out of a sense of uncertainty had generated its own news stories across North America and ended up snowballing as a result. Grocery stores, pharmacies, and retailers assured us that supply chains were strong but that restocking each day was a challenge, one that led to the appearance of scarcity.

In my now-daily early morning call with the leaders from not only health but other key ministries, we discussed options. At one point I expressed my concern that the public health emergency I'd declared lacked provisions to support municipalities. During the 2009 H1N1 pandemic I'd seen how important this issue was: when a vaccine had become available, we'd had trouble establishing mass immunization clinics simply because municipalities had no way to access the funds needed to use municipal buildings, community centres, and schools for vaccinating people. And that was just one example of the kinds of problems we'd faced. So for the last ten years I'd been advocating to have complementary provisions in B.C.'s Public Health Act and Emergency Management Act to ensure a broad all-government response when we needed it. Now, of course, such advocacy had been overtaken by this emergency—and we were still dealing with competing legislation at different levels of government.

In addition, municipal and regional governments were now wanting to introduce different and sometimes contradictory measures to address the pandemic—from fining people who were standing too close in public places to mandating mask wearing. My concern was that this would create a hodgepodge approach across the province, one that would not only undermine public support but also lead to inequities. It wasn't lost on me that whenever fines and enforcement measures were implemented, racialized and impoverished people suffered more. Far better, in my mind, to develop a single, coherent response that relied on communication and common suffering rather than shaming or fines.

In our phone call that morning, as we talked through the Emergency Management Act provisions, we came to the conclusion that a unified approach would accomplish many helpful things, among them these two: the management of scarce resources (thus solving our toilet paper crisis) and the superseding of municipal bylaws.

That very afternoon, the minister of public safety declared a provincial state of emergency—one that would assist in supporting not only the public health and health system response, but also municipal governments in a coherent, coordinated response across British Columbia. And just as I'd planned during my short flight across the water, my address at our media appearance later in the day focused on hope: on reminding people that we still had cherry blossoms and mountains, and that now more than ever we needed to hug the children in our lives and hold our families close—whomever we might consider family.

I also felt strongly that we needed to give people the release of going outdoors, to grant them permission to go out and play. I knew, from the empirical evidence, that outside was better than inside for avoiding any respiratory virus, and that being out in the fresh air conferred both mental and physical health benefits. So I started a daily call for people to go for a walk while keeping a safe distance from others—to take their family, their pets, their children, or just themselves outside each day, even for a few minutes. Move meetings or coffee dates or grandparent visits outside, I suggested. And I called on cities and towns across the province to make this easier by designating streets or lanes or parks for the people, a way to give everyone the chance for some air and (when it appeared on our rainy coast) sun.

LATE THAT AFTERNOON, after the briefing, I was walking the deserted streets back to my hotel when a message came in from my team: the federal government had implemented travel restrictions under the Quarantine Act. This would mandate, finally, that anyone returning to Canada from outside the country must quarantine for fourteen days or risk federal penalties up to $750,000. At the same time, the prime minister had appealed to those Canadians still abroad to "come home." So far, the federal government hadn't had the resources to enforce or even monitor quarantine restrictions. Although we'd been appealing for weeks for such action, setting up a system that would actually work would be a challenge. Suddenly I felt exhausted again. I believed it was the right call, but the prospect of managing thousands of Canadians coming home—and bringing the risk of COVID-19 with them—was daunting.

My hotel felt ghostly and empty, with only a skeleton staff remaining. The restaurant and bar were now closed, as were all the luxury shops in the normally bustling lobby. I was one of only twenty or so guests in a hotel whose more than five hundred rooms were normally full. They still had room service, though, so I settled into a lovely suite on the thirteenth floor with space to work and a view of the harbour, the Olympic

Plaza in the distance. The events of the next few hours would imprint that room in my memory for a long time.

After finally wrapping up my emails and teleconferences, I fell into the comfortable king-size bed around eleven, my now ever-present thoughts and worries racing through my mind. Hours later, around four thirty, I was jolted awake by the fire alarm. I'd been roused from sleep by a hotel fire alarm before, but this was different: I smelled smoke. Not a false alarm, then. Fully awake now, I reached for my shoes and jacket as the manager's voice came over the intercom advising everyone to "evacuate immediately."

I stuffed my computer, wallet, and iPhone into my bag and headed out into the empty hallway; I was the only guest on the floor. I made my way to the nearest stairway and started down. Disconcertingly, the staircase was also deserted; I could smell smoke and hear the alarm, but nothing else. Three floors down the staircase came to an abrupt end, forcing me to enter the hallway and find another way out. This was the beauty of eccentric old buildings and why I loved this hotel, but that early morning it was making me more and more anxious.

Finally I found another staircase and continued down. It, too, was empty and seemed endless, but eventually I emerged through a back door into the alley behind the hotel. Still not another soul in sight. I could hear sirens, though, so I strode, heart racing, around to the driveway entrance. No one. I was looking around, dazed and uncertain, when a staff person rounded the corner and called out to me. "Oh, good!" she said. "We're all on the other side. Come with me."

I walked with her, full of gratitude, to the plaza across the street, joining the little cluster there of guests and staff. Someone brought blankets and someone else took roll call: all present and accounted for, if a little shaken. Together, we watched the fire crews do their work.

After what seemed an eternity—the sun was rising now; it was going on six thirty—we were allowed back in the building. It had been a real fire: an electrical short in one of the empty lobby stores. All was well, but there was a strong smell of smoke throughout the building. And although we were given the option of moving to a sister property, I wanted to return to my room: I took comfort in the familiarity of this place despite being rather rattled. I even managed a short half hour of sleep before the day began again.

A COUPLE OF HOURS LATER, walking down the empty city streets to our Vancouver government offices, again I felt weary. The intensity of the past weeks and the gravity of the measures we'd taken weighed on me. No doubt the fire alarm hadn't helped—that, and the constant flying back and forth between Victoria and Vancouver. I was feeling more and more disconnected from my team, and worried I was missing important signals. I was also missing the essential conversations I'd been having with the deputy minister in Victoria, ones in which we'd work through the possibilities and our options for action.

As the communications team convened in the rooms overlooking the harbour, settling in to develop the plan for the day, I could tell they were tired, too. Like me, they'd been alternating between camping out in these offices and the ones in Victoria. We were all feeling nomadic and displaced, and the pressure and scrutiny we were under only increased the intensity.

Even so, as I looked around the room my mood lifted a little; I couldn't help smiling. We were a ragtag group, with a variety of complementary skills: government communications employees, ministerial assistants, and a private communications expert to help with my messages and media commitments. I felt incredibly lucky to have them all.

It hadn't always been this way. The Ministry of Health's overall portfolio was so broad and complex that initially I'd been somewhat on my own, with only a skeleton crew. When the pandemic began, one person had been quickly assigned to public health specifically, but with all the issues we managed, they were on a steep learning curve. Then, as things heated up in January, a communications lead had been assigned for my office, but they, too, were rapidly overwhelmed. Recognizing that it was only going to get busier, I had asked—begged, really—for help.

That had come in the form of a senior communications expert who ran her own company in Vancouver. As soon as she joined the team, I was able to breathe again. She triaged media requests, which were coming fast and furious, and worked with both the minister's office and the government communications people—an imaginative, thoughtful, inventive group— so that we could all coordinate. By March we'd developed a daily cadence, beginning with an early morning teleconference (or occasionally some of us would meet in person) to run through the day and develop the themes for our media statement. We'd also discuss the things the minister and I would need to bring up in the live media briefing.

It was this fabulous team that came up with many of the mantras we would eventually use, and it was through bouncing words off them that I'd developed my key counsel: be kind, be calm, be safe. I may have formulated it, and I certainly spoke it aloud in my own way, but they were able to pick up on its resonance and amplify it—and remind me to say it regularly.

Still, by mid-March we were all flagging. And so later that day, between the provincial and national calls, I had a talk with the minister and deputy. We needed to pull back and regroup. With the measures we'd put in place, and now the federal edict to "stay home"—reinforcing our own state of provincial emergency and "work from home" message—it was time to stop the back and forth. We all agreed that, for the foreseeable future, Saturday would be our last Vancouver media briefing. We would reconvene in Victoria and only the minister would travel, coming over once weekly.

After our regular briefing that day, the minister and I held the first of what would become regular town hall sessions. For an hour on live TV, we answered questions from the hosts and from the people of B.C., who emailed, videoed, and wrote in. These town halls would soon evolve into an important way to talk directly to the public about wide-ranging issues. That first time, though, was the most stressful for me, not knowing what would be asked or how the format would be received. And it was exhausting—my tiredness compounded by my previous night's adventures. But by the end I felt pleased. Here was a chance to answer so many of the nagging questions people had: Did we really mean work from home, what was physical distancing, how do you wash your hands, do masks work, do I need to sanitize boxes delivered to my house? At that time, too, we were still adjusting to the reality of the risk of cruises and air travel. On this I was unequivocal: cruises and international travel were to be avoided for now. And if you did go, yes, you must isolate for fourteen days when you return; that was an order and non-negotiable. I can still hear and see the expressions of disbelief that we were really going to do this, that we were serious.

—

THE OMINOUS FEELING in the air closed back in on me as I returned to my hotel in the evening dark. This would be its last night open; its remaining crew were shutting things down. Most staff had been laid off for the time being—and the anxiety was painfully evident in every face. No one, least of all me, knew how long this would last, or what the world would look like if and when it was over.

I had dinner from the limited room-service menu as my calls went late into the night—although I could hardly complain; for my East Coast colleagues it was well past midnight. The federal government was weighing its options, watching cases climb in Ontario and Quebec as well as in B.C. It was apparent that the pandemic in central Canada was intensifying dramatically and that measures needed to be taken quickly.

Meanwhile, with tens of thousands still crossing land and air borders into Canada daily, imported cases continued to drive the rapid increases we were seeing, along with their spillover into communities across the country. Only essential travel was now permitted, in effect closing our borders with the world and, most significantly, our long undefended border with the United States, our largest trading partner. And since similar measures were being taken internationally, putting travellers in danger of being stranded, the prime minister continued to implore Canadians everywhere to come home. The repatriation flights the government had started arranging in China were also continuing, but worldwide travel was screeching to a halt and commercial flights were being cancelled. It was becoming clear that there was no way the government could rescue every single Canadian abroad.

During my calls I heard how every province and territory was bracing for the influx, knowing the federal resources at our borders would be woefully inadequate for monitoring everyone coming in. This migration was driven by businesses bringing staff back, students returning as schools and universities shuttered, and people losing their jobs around the world as cities and countries locked down. For many Canadians, this return also meant leaving homes where they'd lived for years. Yet the need to be closer to family and community in a crisis was strong, especially for those returning from the U.S. And it was apparent to me, as it was to my colleagues across the country, that some would be bringing the virus home with them, too. We needed to be prepared.

On Saturday morning, after another fitful sleep (mercifully uninterrupted by fire alarms), I got up for an early call with the WHO on mass gatherings. Then it was time to leave the hotel. As I was checking out, the staff gathered round and kindly gave me a hamper filled with food, teas and coffee, and a beautiful cake; they were packing up the kitchen and thought I should take some of the perishables to get me through the days ahead. We said a sad, subdued goodbye in the near-deserted lobby, all of us wishing for a time when the storm had passed.

Unspoken was our fear of just how bad that storm might be. I was reminded of the words of Maya Angelou: "Every storm runs out of rain." If only I knew whether our emergency measures would hold before that happened.

IN LYNN HENRY'S WORDS

On Thursday, March 19—no longer a Thursday at all like any other, a Thursday after the Wednesday when the province of British Columbia declared a state of emergency—I woke early in the dark, alone and cold (it was a running joke that there were never quite enough quilts on the spare-room bed) in my sister's house. My phone on the side table was buzzing. I turned it over and squinted at the screen. Five thirty-five a.m. The sound of a whoosh, and there was a selfie from Bonnie. Her face, with a part-amused, part-chagrined expression, peered out from under a thick yellow blanket. In the background: dark office towers, the flash of red and orange lights, one spindly tree in a deserted public square, ghost-grey streets. *This is how my morning started*, the bubble of her message read.

Rewind to the day before: my younger sister, nephew, and niece had flown in a half-empty plane back across the closing-down country even as Bonnie had made her regular Helijet hop to Vancouver for the end-of-week press briefings with the health minister. She'd return home late Saturday afternoon, and the week's cycle of phone calls, meetings and briefings, dizzying news, heart-stopping numbers, and above all people's lives changing in both fast and slow motion would begin again.

Having made the pact to stay put just as my two sisters scattered, I felt simultaneously released and unmoored from every familiar rhythm in my life. (Later, thinking back, I realized this was also when I first felt a thrum of puzzling heartbreak start up, a chord of constant mourning that for months would underlie every experience, even—or especially—glancing moments of delight or happiness. For a while, it mildly distressed me: How was I suffering? I couldn't yet see how painfully small my orbit was, how explosively our new universe was expanding, how atomized its essential matter would become once its constituent parts were separated and exposed—sometimes violently— by COVID-size distance.) So, after watching Bonnie hurry off to her helicopter ride in the shadows and drizzle of early morning Wednesday, I'd booted up my computer and set myself on a new regimen: dial into work, remotely, from seven a.m. until about two or three p.m., which synced up nicely with Toronto and New York, three hours ahead; then go out and walk about the neighbourhood for a couple of hours, doing necessary errands along the way, and witnessing, in a semi-daze like so many others I spotted on their own strolls, the continually morphing customs of our strange new world.

Over the following days I would tune into the health minister's and Bonnie's COVID briefings at three p.m., wherever I happened to be: sometimes still working at Bonnie's kitchen table, but often from a place in the park or along the seawall path where I'd notice others doing the same, fixed on their phones, pressing hands to headsets, still as statues on benches or rocky outcrops for the hour-long broadcast, and sometimes observed quizzically (or was this my imagination?) by birds and squirrels and other small animals in the underbrush. Perhaps the creatures who circled our human lives sensed a change, some new syncopation with consequences yet to be lived through—although to a human older than, say, forty, the unmissable broadcasts were improbably old-fashioned: how curious it was, to return to an era when a good portion of the people in a community would tune into one newscast at an appointed time to hear portents of our collective fate.

Although I mostly listened to the briefings on the radio, I could picture their backdrop clearly. In fact, to rewind twenty-four hours further, to Tuesday the 17th, Bonnie had invited me to observe the daily COVID conference in person at the legislature while Sarah and the teenagers ran errands on what would be their last day in the west. In the brightness of that early afternoon, around one p.m., I had watched from the legislature steps as Bonnie walked along Government Street, past an unnaturally quiet inner harbour, its buskers vanished and boats moored, bare masts gently swaying, and crossed onto the green cut grass of the parliament building grounds. I raised my hand in greeting and she caught up with me, then led us both round the building to a side entrance tucked into a grand, stone-pillared walkway that looked out over the sturdy back of a statue of Queen Victoria and a perfect city view. An extraordinary totem pole, anchored incongruously in cement but seeming to have grown up from hidden roots under the manicured lawn, stood in the corner of the view, at a contemplative angle to both queen and town. Bonnie waved her access card, the heavy door swung open, and we clipped along an otherwise deserted, gleaming corridor lined on one side with the faces of men, mostly, in identical dark brown frames, and on the other side with the delicate pastels of stained glass lit by spring sun.

A lone security guard nodded courteously at us as we climbed a set of wide marble stairs and arrived outside a locked wooden door. Pinned to it was a large piece of paper with COVID-19 hygiene protocols and warnings in urgent red ink. Bonnie rapped quickly on the door and slipped inside as it opened, and I followed, swiping my hands under the waiting liquid sanitizer. "Hello, hello," she said, hanging her coat on a hook and extending her hand for mine. "This is my sister Lynn. She's going to be our audience today."

We'd entered the spacious, high-ceilinged central room in the suite of offices inhabited by the minister of health and his hardworking, mostly (to my eye) youthful staff. Five faces, spaced carefully at appropriate distances around the room, looked up briefly, nodded and smiled, and turned back to their work. A woman's head poked out of a small office beside a galley kitchen to say a curious hello. "Help yourself to coffee," she said. "Although I'm afraid I can't vouch for it." She nodded at a closed door on the opposite side of the common space and said to Bonnie, "The minister's just on a call. He'll be ready in a couple of minutes."

An affable, well-spoken young man who introduced himself as the ministry's senior communications officer placed a sheaf of papers on a table and then stepped politely away to a safe distance. "The printout of the numbers," he said. "And what we're thinking for today's release." Bonnie reached for the report and gave it a sharp-eyed scan. These were the daily figures detailing confirmed COVID infections, compiled by scientists at the B.C. Centre for Disease Control from each of the five regional health authorities in the five geographical areas of the province. (Their system worked this way: local doctors or health practitioners sent notice of any testing to the regional authority, who then relayed numbers daily to the Centre, who collated and analyzed them and produced the document Bonnie saw.) The report was also seen by the First Nations Health Authority and the Deputy Provincial Health Officer for Indigenous Health—led by two accomplished First Nations physicians whom Bonnie relied on and consulted regularly. "I saw the numbers earlier this morning back at my office, and talked them through with the MHOS [medical health officers]," my sister explained to me, glancing up, "but I always get them printed out here so that the minister and I can review and have them on hand."

The door to the inner office opened abruptly, and Minister Dix—bespectacled, slim, suit-and-tied, around the same age as my sister, I guessed; charged with a crackle of energy and curiosity—stepped into the main space. "Come in, come in," he insisted genially after we were introduced, and so before the door closed again I slid quietly into the chair closest to Bonnie and most distant from everyone else, joining them both at a big oval wooden worktable in his room. The young woman who'd earlier said hello—the minister's senior ministerial assistant, it turned out—came in, too, perching with papers and notebook on a sofa against the far wall. I glanced up at the clock over the door: forty-five minutes to go before the briefing in front of the cameras.

I listened as the minister and Bonnie went rapidly through the numbers and discussed their respective talking points. As with the phone conversation I'd overheard days earlier between my sister and the deputy minister, I was struck by the brisk, collegial shorthand of their dialogue, although now there was also a structure to the exchange, clearly familiar to both participants in these pre-press sessions (it faintly reminded me of Aaron Sorkin–style patter), along with an odd top note of anticipation and nerves. I wondered about this seeming anxiety; by now, in a feat of public speaking that was both astonishing and unimaginable to me, Bonnie and the minister, sometimes led by the premier, had delivered almost fifty such presentations in a row. The protocol for delivering the data itself was like a familiar refrain: new cases; unwelcome deaths; hospitalizations; recoveries. These raw figures were then broken down for the press by geographical region, by health authority.

During the live briefings, as I would soon witness, this essential recitation was followed by an equally important pause: first my sister, in her way, and then the minister, in his way, would express their condolences for those we had lost. Indeed, something I admired about the minister that day—and came to admire more over time as the numbing numbers were tallied and as I watched others, in other places and in other ways, day after day deliver their own figures to the press and the people— to you and I, to all of *us*—was his matter-of-fact yet unwavering insistence on acknowledging the humans behind the facts, and by extension their connection to layers upon layers of people (starting with family, friends, and caregivers and rippling out from there), their indelible and singular stories.

But in the minister's office that Tuesday, it began to dawn on me that I might be about to observe no ordinary briefing. "Are you ready?" the minister was saying pointedly to Bonnie. "Are *we* ready?" This was phrased as a question, but his tone suggested no hesitation. *I support this; we will do this*, it said.

I thought back to what Bonnie had told me the previous evening, over a nightcap, about the background to that particular day's startling news: it was the Monday when Prime Minister Trudeau had announced the federal government's intention to close our country's borders to non-essential travellers who did not hold Canadian citizenship; the Monday when British Columbia was urging its citizens not to travel internationally for March break and putting in place mandatory quarantine orders for those who did. (It was also the Monday when Bonnie had apologetically but decisively given our sister Sarah and her children their hastily changed tickets back to PEI.)

"Why these measures right now?" I'd asked her then. "I mean, I think I understand in the larger context. I see what's happening in Italy. I get that the cruise ships are a potential disaster and at the very least a worry. But what exactly tipped us this way today?"

Bonnie sipped her drink thoughtfully. Then suddenly she got up from her blue velvet chair, opened the kitchen door to the back stoop, and stepped outside into the still night. "Aha!" she exclaimed. "I almost forgot." She came back in smiling triumphantly, holding a large bag filled with carefully piled recyclable containers. Inside were home-cooked meals for the week and a lovely little bouquet of wildflowers. A colleague on maternity leave, Bonnie explained as she stored the food away, and the colleague's mother prepared a weekly offering for her now, knowing how little time she had to cook. I peered out the back door before locking it for the night and noticed a trace of something unusual on the steps there. I flicked on the porch light—and the curve of a chalk rainbow materialized on the top step, with the words *Thank You* gleaming faintly in grey-blue one step below. A chalky pink heart separated the *Thank* and the *You*.

Bonnie had settled back in her chair. She was exhausted, of course, and looked wan even under the soft warmth of her living-room lamp, but I could see that the terrible, all-consuming dread and stress of the weekend had subsided a little, now that the day's extraordinary announcements about travel had been made. "So, to answer your question," she said. "Yes, there were a number of things that combined to make a perfect virus storm. First, that day you arrived last week—March 12, I think, right? . . . Well, that morning I had one of my regular conversations with my colleagues in Washington State, and they told me, 'It's everywhere here.' Which meant the virus had to be spreading in B.C., too, beyond the cases we already knew about, which could be traced back to China or, in one new case I was following, Iran. We did some genome sequencing of new cases here and found that indeed it was the same or similar to the strain in Washington. That meant, without a doubt, that community spread was happening, and that we now had a number of different, geographically unrelated strains circulating."

She sighed. "And then there's the international dentists' conference in Vancouver that somehow went ahead despite all the public health warnings. Fifteen thousand people from around the world, Lynn." Bonnie let that sink in for a moment. "Anyhow—at first I was told that the only case of COVID-19 there involved one dentist who was at the conference for only two hours, someone who'd gone to a conference in Munich directly beforehand. So, of course, we quickly did the contact tracing and testing, and realized through those efforts and in talking to people that much more of the virus was circulating than could be traced back to that one infected person. So I issued an order: anyone who'd been at the conference needed to go home, isolate for two weeks, monitor their health, and close their practice. Not a popular order," Bonnie added ruefully. "And there was some resistance. But what I tried to tell people is that we all have a vested interest in getting this right—for the sake of everyone's health, but also for our collective lives in every way, social, economic, cultural. Psychological, even."

My sister stood again, retrieved her phone from where she'd left it on the kitchen table, and sat back down, restlessly and expertly scrolling through the hundred or so new unread messages that had popped into her inbox in the twenty minutes since she had poured our drinks, occasionally murmuring "What??" or "Oh, that gives me a bit of hope." She still diligently read, I knew, every message, and responded to a staggering number. It would be a couple more weeks before her office, overwhelmed, crafted an automatic reply that gave Bonnie and her small team at least the illusion of a pause during which they might reasonably answer.

"I guess there are probably two other factors that led to the announcements today, and the ones that will follow soon," she continued, without looking up from the screen. "I think I already told you about Quebec, how they had their March break a couple of weeks ago, which meant we have this little window in which we're seeing infection in travellers returning home, especially from France. We've been discussing that in our national Special Advisory Committee, with all the chief public health officers, over the past several days. And then, too, I simply believe that we're at the tipping point now with the spread in the community—the different strains now circulating; knowing that many people were about to travel for the break; understanding a little more clearly who is vulnerable, and by that I mean particularly the elders in our community, all those grandparents, for example, who might be exposed through travel themselves or returning family.

"And, of course, the overarching goal, the thing that underpins everything we do in this moment, is to keep this manageable and not overwhelm our hospitals all at once, like we've seen in other places in the world, unfortunately. You know, for months now I've known the specifics of every single positive case of this virus here in our province, and all the contacts each person had, but recently we reached a point where that just isn't possible.

"And there's another event that pushed me further along this path: we had a positive test in a person who's been in the hospital for other reasons for about ninety days. So this is worrisome. It means the virus came along with either a visitor or someone inside the hospital already, who may not know they have the virus. And again, this means it's circulating in ways we can no longer completely contain. The time is right now to take this seriously as a community and put protective measures in place—most particularly for healthcare workers and vulnerable people."

Bonnie looked up from her phone at last, then placed it face down on her side table, its pale pink case glinting. She swirled and finished the last mouthful of her nightcap, set the glass down firmly too, and looked at me. "What I'm about to tell you is a huge deal, because it gives me the responsibility and power to issue enforceable orders, verbally as well as in writing . . . But here goes: for about a week, the government and I have been talking about possibly declaring a public health emergency."

On Tuesday afternoon, as the clock ticked evenly in the minister's office, these remembered words were like a siren of subtext for the seemingly straightforward exchange I was hearing.

"Tomorrow in Vancouver, then," the minister was saying, "after your public health declaration today, our government will announce a provincial state of emergency, along with the new orders for entertainment, restaurants, cafés, schools." He rose from the table, went over to his expansive desk under the far windows, and clicked the keyboard on his computer, gazing at its screen. Then he said, "I'm worried about all the people whose elective surgery will have to be cancelled or delayed."

Bonnie nodded. "I know," she said quietly. "I know there are people who are suffering. We just need to think of it as doing what we have to do now so that we can reopen soon, with as little pain to go around as possible." She returned to her notes, marking a few changes here and there in pen. "Okay. I really am ready," she said a few moments later.

"Where are we?" the minister said, looking up at the clock. Two minutes to three. "All right. Shall we go?" He opened the door and led the way out of his chambers, Bonnie following after a six-foot pause, gesturing at me to join them. We clipped along in our little formation—Bonnie and the minister volleying quick questions and answers into the space between them—back down the winding staircase, along an airy arched hallway, and again down a narrower, older, more cramped and half-lit set of stairs until we emerged at the door to a concrete underground tunnel, ribbons of pipes stretching overhead like the rorqual grooves of a whale's underbelly. At the far mouth of the tunnel: the small, windowless, press-briefing amphitheatre, its bank of cameras already on, a row of sparkling white teeth. As we passed security in the tunnel, one of the guards holding open the door gave Bonnie and the minister a small nod. "You're doing a great job for us," he said. "Thank you."

Inside the cramped theatre, a smattering of journalists sat in separate rows at carefully staggered intervals while others dialed in by phone. (I would attend three such briefings during my visit, and this was the only one where I saw even a small handful of reporters in person; each time the number of people in the room would dwindle until finally there were only cameras, the person deftly handling the phone, and the mesmerizing sign-language interpreter—a fixture at the press conferences who soon became so popular that he had his own fan club.) The minister spoke first, acknowledging the land and its First Peoples before introducing Bonnie. The now-familiar recitation of numbers began, and sombre condolences were expressed for the people who had died, in that moment still less than ten, which paradoxically made each single blow seem all the more painful—*our* citizens, *our* families, *our* loss. Then Bonnie took a breath, and in her low, steady tone explained and declared a public health emergency in the province, effective immediately. Into the startled pause that followed, she leaned forward and enunciated, for the first time, the full phrase whose bits and pieces had been combining and recombining in her speech for weeks: "This is our time to be kind, to be calm, and to be safe."

Although the words were careful and deliberate and engineered to stick in people's minds, I suspect my sister could not have known that, once out in the air, this sentence—its theme and variations—would almost instantly spread, evolving into cards, buttons, bags, T-shirts, face masks, candles, needlepoint sayings, paintings, quilts, hooked rugs, headlines, posters, editorial cartoons, bracelets, pendants, paperweights, cookies, hoodies, coffee cups, billboards. (Months later, on one of the small Gulf Islands of the Salish Sea, as I hiked on a hot day along a dirt footpath through the woods, I would spot a series of smooth, bright-painted rocks, half-hidden under expansively shrugging ferns and nestled in the roots of massive trees, bearing the sweetly decorated suggestions *Be Kind* and *Stay Safe*; still later, on a twisting mountain road that dropped to a deep-blue bay, I would pass a hand-lettered plea on a piece of faded pink construction paper attached to a crossroads' light pole: *BE KIND. BE CALM. BE SAFE. DR. BONNIE.*)

THE JARRING JUMBLE of the past two days' events—especially the two states of emergency, public health and provincial, falling like dominoes one after the other on Tuesday and Wednesday, and who knew where the chain would end?— crowded my mind as I blinked at the photo from Bonnie that had lit up my phone early Thursday morning. "What is going on?" I typed. "You okay?"

"I am sitting out in the square by the Vancouver Art Gallery, waiting for the fire service to do their thing," she texted back. "There was a fire in one of the shops on the ground floor of my hotel, and the alarm went off and we had to evacuate." Another swoosh and a new photo arrived, this time a streetscape with even more red and yellow flashes reflecting off tall dark buildings.

I reached for my glasses and peered more closely at the image. Despite the splotches of bright colour and the fire truck, its massive grey ladders folded like wings, in the centre of the scene, the area around the hotel looked deserted—except for my sister and a single firefighter in full gear. "Have you been out there for long?" I wrote. "Weird that you seem like the only patron of the hotel . . ."

"About half an hour," Bonnie texted. "We are going back in soon. Lots of smoke but the fire was small." There was a pause, then: "Yeah, there are about twenty of us in the entire hotel, including staff. Going in now. Will try to catch an hour of sleep. Xx."

I put my phone on the bedside table and imagined my sister's hours ahead after that early little conflagration. No doubt, I decided, it would be the least troubling and stressful part of the day: momentarily difficult, sure, but out of her control and resolvable by others. I lay in the freezing dark for a minute or two longer, listening to the relentless morning screels and caws of the neighbourhood's seagulls and crows, and for the first time felt utterly undone, small and solitary and afraid.

The day, however, once it arrived in full, turned out to be heedlessly gorgeous, and so that afternoon, after work at the kitchen table and phone calls and Zoom meetings, I wandered out into the park and stationed myself on a bench to stream the COVID briefing on my phone. I watched Bonnie step up to the lectern, poised and serious, not a puff of smoke to be seen. The City of Vancouver declared its own state of emergency, in step now with the province. The B.C. courts were to close. The prime minister in Ottawa had announced the stunning shutdown of the border between Canada and the United States, which in B.C. would affect travel to and from Washington State. Bonnie and the health minister reinforced the public health order to close all bars and restaurants and for these businesses to move towards providing takeout meals only. And they acknowledged one more death, part of an outbreak at the Lynn Valley Care Centre, bringing British Columbia's total count to a wrenching eight.

"Physical distancing is not optional," Bonnie said firmly near the end of the hour, before moving back from the microphone and carefully out of camera range.

I looked up at last from my tiny, weightless screen with its enormous, crushing news. I was sitting in an interior part of the park I had somehow never noticed before, its edges marked by high trees with softly rustling leaves at one end and a gently curving semicircle of newly blooming shrubbery at the other, giving it the feel of a private walled garden. A young couple directly across from me were exclaiming as they watched their toddler daughter take a few steps on the bright green grass towards a seemingly unconcerned duck. To one side, an older woman in a wide-brimmed, cone-shaped straw hat sat with her eyes closed on a sun-dappled bench beside a bed of tulips. It was an astonishingly, absurdly bucolic tableau, stillness at the centre of a cyclone, and despite myself I felt an almost euphoric rush. This had something to do, I supposed, with the simple normalcy of the scene coupled with the knowledge that, at least for now and in the foreseeable time to come, our ways of being with and around people—strangers and friends alike—had radically changed. Indeed, in our physically distant world, a close friend was to be kept as far away as the woman daydreaming on the bench, the child tripping across the grass. Yet for a minute— a minute that even as it occurred felt fleeting—there we were, five strangers randomly and companionably enjoying a spring-time garden together.

I strolled away and back home down the slope of a hill, the warmth and euphoria trailing away. It was a curious thing, though: from time to time over the following two weeks, until the day I left town, I retraced my steps and searched, befuddled, but found I could never quite wind my way back to that exact place in the park again. And already the darker green and brown-leaf edges of this entire patch of ground between the town and the sea had begun to shift and evolve: striding through the field of feathery wild grasses closest to my sister's house, I saw that two small tents had planted themselves side by side, just far enough into the first ring of trees to be barely visible from the busy road. A young woman in shorts, T-shirt, and boots sat inside one, reading a paperback book, ignoring passersby.

That night, on a quick call to close what must have been one of the longest among a series of endless days, Bonnie said, uncharacteristically and with hesitation, "I'm still worried people don't get social distancing. I'm thinking . . . should I put more controls in place?" I knew my sister was musing aloud, not really asking me, but still I was startled.

"I don't know," I replied, truthfully.

"I saw some tents in the park today," I ventured a moment later. "People are taking refuge there, I think."

"Ah yes," Bonnie said, her tone brightening. "Yes. I know. Actually, the government is working on a plan with the cities and the shelters and a bunch of other organizations that, I hope, I believe, might make a difference for street-involved people with regard to safer housing. This is the time to do it, if ever there was a time. So we shall see. I can tell you more about what I know when I'm home."

THE NEXT DAY, FRIDAY, on my mid-afternoon walk, I spotted another single tent pitched even farther inside the perimeter of the park, a pair of resident peacocks jerkily marching past its zipped-up entry. In contrast, just across busy Dallas Road that marked the edge of the park, and down past the cliffs on the beach, I passed groups of families gathering happily on long tusks of driftwood for picnics, and a huddle of a dozen young men and women, cold drinks stashed in a cooler by the cliff, playing a joyous, back-clapping game of volleyball.

I thought of my sister's halting, agonized question of the night before. And I recalled words I had heard on the radio that very morning; I had paused in my work to listen because I recognized the voice. Gentle and considered and intelligent, it belonged to an author I publish, Madeleine Thien. She had been asked by the host how a writer might think about the moment we were living through. "I say to my students," Maddie replied, "do you really want to spend the next five years reading novels about the pandemic?" She gave the awfulness of that possibility a moment of pointed silence. Then she continued: "I say to them, and to everyone, it is incredibly important instead to examine the ground we're standing on, and what led up to here."

As I circled back towards home, I went by one of the handful of seniors' residences overlooking the beach and its mirage-like view of faraway mountains on the other side of the water. A number of its street-facing windows displayed cut-outs of big red hearts, and two banners had been draped prominently above its entrance: *Thank You, Healthcare Workers!* and *Thank You, Dr. Bonnie!* The building looked quite locked up, though, and the U-shaped drive leading to its front door (which even from a distance I could see was covered in notices and warnings) was empty of cars or visitors or the usual residents with canes and walkers, with the exception of two weary-looking women in their thirties, I guessed, walking purposefully towards the entryway in nurses' uniforms. Along the side of the building, an elderly woman sat alone in a wheelchair on her fifth-floor balcony and waved at me when I looked up. I waved back, my heart constricting, thinking of my own parents safe still (I hoped) in their own home, far away beside another sea.

"You know," I texted my sister as I neared home. "Re: your question of last evening. I think the answer is, maybe you do.

Need more clarity, I mean, about distancing. You would know best about all the implications, and who really suffers. But, maybe . . . ?"

What I did not know then was that Bonnie had already received a letter from a group of hospital emergency and critical care doctors urging her to implement stronger and more stringent lockdown measures. She would reply three days later, on Sunday, March 22, calmly detailing how everything being called for had already been imposed but refusing to attach harsher or more punitive language or consequences to her orders. Her consistent, unshakable reasoning during this time was that, if provided clear scientific evidence and direction, most people would comply with what was being asked of them. And her constant concern, even while balancing in her mind and heart the legitimate worries of her fellow physicians, was that those who were already disadvantaged in society would be more harshly affected by harsher ways.

That response was still slightly in the future, though, when I walked out along the seawall towards the Helijet terminal in Saturday's mid-afternoon sun. Bonnie emerged from its tiny hut as I arrived, wearing her light pink plaid overcoat and laden down with an impossible number of shoulder bags. "Hello. What's all this?" I asked.

"Well, it turns out I'll be the last patron in the hotel for the time being. They're shutting down for now. So they wanted me to take a bunch of stuff with me—mostly tea and biscuits and chocolate. We'll have a small feast."

I shouldered a brimming bag and we strode along the seawall path home, Bonnie wheeling her little suitcase behind her, patent-leather shoes flashing cheerfully in the sun. "Also," she said, "the minister and I decided that we should no longer travel back and forth between Vancouver and Victoria. There can't be any non-essential trips right now. I'll work from here while he and much of his office remain over there."

A car passing us slowed, and a man leaned out the passenger-side window. "Hey, Dr. Bonnie Henry," he called. "Thank you for everything you're doing!" A little farther along we stepped aside to let an older couple stroll by at a safe distance. They both smiled in recognition. "You're doing such a good job," one said.

Bonnie smiled in return and clasped her hands together in a little salute of thanks. I knew she felt a terrifying mix of emotion over this increasing public acknowledgment: shyness, diffidence, self-deprecation, extreme embarrassment. But I intuited that she'd also begun to create a Dr. Bonnie persona, slightly apart from her private self, that allowed her to accept these now inevitable interactions with grace—even, in some circumstances, allowing herself a grain of pleasure.

"Hey, that's rather sweet," I said encouragingly.

"Oh, it's all fine and good until the public inquiries and class-action lawsuits begin," she said wryly. "This is not my first pandemic, you know."

"Well then, welcome back to your bubble for good." I opened my arms in a mock embrace.

Bonnie laughed. "I'm going to miss you when you're gone," she said, emphasis on *gone*, and gave me a half-joking half smile.

PART III

BE SAFE

{ Weeks Three and Four: March into April }

IN DR. BONNIE HENRY'S WORDS

Across the province, and indeed the country, we were moving home: working from home, learning from home, retreating into our household bubbles, battening down the hatches, and waiting. It felt to me as if we were collectively holding our breath, even as hospitalizations climbed and more and more people needed intensive care. These were what we called lag indicators: it was two or three weeks after case numbers rose before hospitalizations, too, started to increase. In some cities we'd seen this happen rapidly, but that was mostly because cases had gone unnoticed until too late.

I knew we needed to focus on bending the curve in our communities while making sure we had the resources—in people and in PPE, in ventilators and in beds—to manage the hospital surge. As the surge started later, it would inevitably go on longer, meaning there would be more transmission and we would have to care for patients for many more weeks. So these next two weeks—or one incubation period—would be critical. We needed to do everything we could to stop transmission—and we needed to do it right now.

Just like me and my colleagues, healthcare workers were watching the global drama unfolding in places like Northern Italy, and they, too, were beginning to feel the effects as our hospital cases grew and more long-term care homes experienced devastating outbreaks. A group of critical care doctors from one hospital publicly called on me to do more and do it fast. They wanted a "complete" lockdown of all services in the province. This was the type of response we'd seen in Hubei and in Northern Italy, where people were forced to stay home except for essential visits to pharmacies, for medical care, and, once a week, for groceries. In some places even going out for groceries wasn't allowed, with people getting fined for being outside at all.

But I strongly believed that we needed to tailor our response to *our* situation, *our* pandemic. During my last briefing in Vancouver I'd already taken what I considered a dramatic step. We'd been seeing more and more cases in community settings, connected to hair and nail salons, massage parlours, spas, and gyms—places where people were in close contact for periods of time indoors. Although many such businesses were taking measures to screen people, enhance cleaning, and reduce numbers, this virus was proving pernicious. Seemingly healthy people could pass it on, and such close quarters were, of course, dangerous to staff and customers alike. So, on that Saturday before I returned to Victoria, I'd reluctantly realized I would have to order all "personal services settings," as we in public health called them, to be closed effective immediately. The risk was simply too great at this point in our pandemic.

Now I ordered many retail stores closed, along with businesses whose staff couldn't work from home. We also reinforced the takeout-only restrictions on restaurants and pubs. And we established COVID-19 guidelines for any businesses that did stay open. This meant that grocery stores, banks, pharmacies, and hardware stores all needed to put specific measures in place—among them erecting Plexiglas barriers, limiting numbers, increasing cleaning, and making hand-cleaning products available as well as health screening for all staff and customers. It took time, of course, for these measures to be set up and for people to adjust to standing in queues, staying apart from others, and wearing masks.

Still, by allowing businesses that could meet these guidelines to remain open, I'd drawn the line at a much different level than had other jurisdictions across the country. Many activities, from garbage collection to lawn maintenance to construction, continued—even if the way they operated looked dramatically different. I believed these were industries and businesses that were amenable to safety guidelines—and were also necessary to ensure that people could keep on with their lives. New seniors' homes needed to be built so that we'd have a place for elders to go; food-packing plants needed to continue, as did banks and plumbing companies. But all of this was yet another balancing act: I wanted to put in just enough restrictions to stop the virus from spreading rapidly while relying on every person in B.C. to do their part.

Talking to the minister and deputy during this time, I suggested that if we could make it to the Easter long weekend with no rapid escalation of infection (and hopefully the reverse), we might be okay. By then influenza season would be over, meaning less respiratory illness in the community and thus an easier time spotting COVID-19. As well, the weather would be warmer—and maybe, just maybe, we'd get a break from that. Influenza and other coronaviruses were seasonal and thrived in the colder, drier months; it was possible that this coronavirus would be similar. But that wasn't a sure thing by any stretch of the imagination. With so many people still susceptible, it was entirely possible that COVID-19 would continue unabated regardless of the weather conditions.

We were learning as we went with this virus, picking up as much as we could from the countries that had been affected ahead of us. We knew by now that early ICU care could increase survival. There was some promising evidence that antiviral medications like remdesivir and other drugs used for HIV could help. Scant preliminary data suggested that hydroxychloroquine might help, too (which later proved not to be true). Accessing such drugs, however, proved a challenge. It seemed every country in the world was looking for the magic cure, with the U.S. in particular acquiring large supplies of some medications, thereby making them unavailable for the rest of the world.

Our research and clinical teams, the ones I'd brought together early in our response, were now working flat out, sharing data with each other and with colleagues around the world. This sharing of data, along with collaboration on clinical trials and case-management successes, was unprecedented. Yet in late March the unknowns still far outweighed the knowns, and our clinical care for patients infected with the virus remained largely supportive. In short, stopping transmission was the most important thing we could do.

AMID THE DARKNESS of these days were stories of survival that brought some rays of light and hope. The eighty-year-old woman who had acquired the virus on a trip to Egypt and Hong Kong and who walked out of the hospital after spending weeks on a ventilator. The Second World War veteran who'd been infected in his long-term care home but recovered in time for his 102nd birthday. And the young respiratory tech on a ventilator in the very ICU where he worked and where he'd become infected. His colleagues cared for him for weeks, sending messages of hope and love as he struggled, until finally he turned the corner to recovery. As he was wheeled out of the hospital, the ICU staff lined the hallway, filled with balloons and decorations, and cheered.

These stories, though, were superseded by the tragedy of those who did not survive: the man in his forties who was seemingly doing well, isolating in the upper floor of his home, and found dead by his frantic wife one morning when he didn't respond to her calls. We were learning that this virus could affect the blood vessels in the lungs and the heart, and that in some people this could lead to catastrophic blood clots and sudden death.

And our greatest tragedy by far was in our long-term care homes, where the virus thrived.

The hard reality was that the only way to prevent hospitalizations and deaths was to prevent transmission. Once someone was exposed to enough of the virus, there was nothing we could do to prevent them from becoming infected. There was no medication we could give, no vaccine that would stop them from getting sick. It was up to their own immune system to fight the virus.

This is where contact tracing came in, and why it was so important. Contact tracing means that once public health identifies a case, we trace everyone the person has had close contact with, people who may have been exposed during the infectious period. We then support these "contacts" in staying home and away from others during the fourteen-day incubation period. Although there's no way of preventing these people from being infected, we *can* stop them from transmitting the infection to anyone else, and we can also make sure they get the healthcare needed if their illness got worse. This is how we break the chains of transmission and stop the spread. And this, I knew, was what would bend our curve. The next two weeks were key. And we needed to convince everyone in B.C. of that.

The more I thought about how to bring everyone along, the more convinced I became of the need to share more than just daily numbers. We needed to share the epidemiology in greater detail—the who, what, and where of the cases we were seeing. We also needed to share the modelling we were using, both to plan for the health sector and to help us understand how we were progressing. These were our "dynamic compartmental models" that used our own data in British Columbia to understand how transmission was happening and what our reproductive number (Rt, or the number of other people each case transmitted to) was on a periodic basis. We had a strong team of epidemiologists and modellers, most of whom were at the B.C. Centre for Disease Control, and we'd funded them in January to start work on these models, knowing we just might need them. I was thankful for that now.

I was, of course, aware that modelling had become a fraught practice of late, in the global response to this pandemic. In the U.K., the respected leader in infectious-disease modelling at Imperial College had released models showing that hundreds of thousands could die—but that "herd immunity" could be achieved if older people were protected while younger people got infected and developed immunity. This had created a stir, to put it mildly. After all, the conventional thinking was that a novel virus like this would burn quickly into a raging inferno, and that control would be a major challenge. Most other models, meanwhile, used basic information on severe illness and deaths—information that had been taken from the initial experience in Wuhan. These models were particularly frightening, as they reflected a worst-case scenario, one in which intervention wasn't available.

But we knew more now, I believed, and in particular, we had a lab-testing strategy that allowed us a better understanding of who was becoming infected. That had to count for something, especially compared to those early days in China, and even in Washington State and Italy, where testing had been delayed until it was too late. Moreover, I'd seen the value of modelling before, in other circumstances, and knew it could help us understand scenarios and the trajectory of our response. I also knew that we couldn't use it to predict the future any more than we could use our daily horoscope.

We weren't the only ones in Canada developing models to help us understand the pandemic. Several other provinces, along with the federal Public Health Agency, were as well. I had asked our team to collaborate with these others as much as possible. Since then we'd developed a strong consortium with several universities in B.C. to augment the BCCDC team and had linked to colleagues in Ontario in particular. Up until now, however, the models and the outputs—I hesitate to call them "predictions," knowing the limitations—were mostly shared only within the circle of decision makers. I believed that we needed to let the public see them—that if the people of B.C. had the same information as we did, it would build trust and understanding.

Making this case was a challenge. Modelling results had leaked out in another province and led to public outcry and concern. These models had suggested a very high death rate and had forecast that hospitals would be overrun. Now, as I discussed with the minister and deputy the value of a public presentation of the usual data *and* the models, I knew much would depend on my ability to explain both clearly. I was convinced that we had to arm people with information they needed to take the measures we were asking of them: stay home if you can, keep safe distances, clean your hands, and stay away from others if you get sick. This was basic infection prevention—so-called motherhood actions—but they worked, and the stakes were high: we needed everyone to buy in.

AS WE PULLED the modelling and data presentation together, our media briefings continued apace, every day but Sunday. The health minister and I remained united in our thinking: "bending the curve" became our rallying cry, along with the importance of caring and connecting with our fellow travellers in this storm.

The fact that people were returning from other countries, particularly the United States, was now causing a great deal of anxiety in the community. Licence plates from California, Washington, and even Alberta triggered fear, and some people were reacting with angry outbursts and bad behaviour, from yelling at people to "go home" to vandalizing cars and shops. The fear of others bringing in the virus had shifted from the Chinese community to anyone who was from "away." To counter this, I reminded people daily that we didn't know everyone else's story, and that individuals had reasons to travel that might not be immediately apparent—which was part of what I meant when I asked people to be kind, and to see others as part of our larger group. Perhaps the person was a Canadian whose school had shut down in Washington State, or a Canadian from California coming home to care for their ailing mother, or one of the many people in B.C. who work in Alberta while living here. These were all our people, members of our community, and we needed to remember to practise compassion and calm.

The media were also starting to pepper me with questions about businesses failing: Did I know that I was putting restaurants out of business; that hair salons, spas, and barbershops would never recover; and that catering companies, wedding planners, and the hotel and tourism industry would perish because of me?

Although I understood on an intellectual level that it wasn't me who'd caused a lethal new virus to disrupt the world, and that the measures I'd implemented were necessary to keep the well away from the sick, and to avoid overwhelming the health systems in the ways that we were witnessing elsewhere, these questions and accusations weighed heavily on me. After all, I knew well that the measures were taking their toll: rates of anxiety and depression were rising, people were drinking more, and reports of inter-partner and family violence were increasing. Such unintended consequences of the measures we had put in place didn't come as a surprise; we'd seen them before during the 2003 SARS outbreak and the 2009 HINI pandemic. But these were on a different scale now: more wide ranging and deeper. The social fabric, not only of my province but across our country, was being torn apart—and not everyone was affected equally. I knew that women, racialized communities, and those living in poverty would be affected most. That wherever there were inequities, the effects of the pandemic would bite harder.

I deeply believed that, more than anything else, we needed to support people through this crisis, and the most vulnerable most of all. But I also knew that this wasn't directly in my control. In my regular meetings with the premier and his cabinet, my job was to let them know what we needed to do to stop COVID-19, and who would be affected most by these measures. Then it was over to them: their role was to step up and put in place the programs to get us through this crisis.

Indeed, in March, as we implemented the restrictions and closures, and looked to the potential impact of these decisions in the future, both the provincial and federal government came out with programs to support individuals financially. They were a much-needed lifeline.

DURING ALL THIS TIME, nothing weighed on me more than the measures we took to protect long-term care homes and hospitals. No visitors were allowed in either venue, not only to reduce the numbers of people coming in but also to preserve PPE. We were perilously short of N95 respirators, and even the basic surgical masks, gowns, and gloves we needed daily were running short. There was no way people could visit these vulnerable settings safely, without putting healthcare workers at risk. And when, despite the measures we had in place, more outbreaks occurred and more deaths followed, it was time to take broader measures.

The movement of healthcare workers between care homes was clearly a risk—a risk that was rapidly proving too great. In my talks with my public health team, this concern came up repeatedly; I took it to the minister and deputy. We needed to make things right, I said, so that healthcare workers could be employed at only one facility and make a living wage. This was a major policy decision that, if implemented, would completely reorganize how we provided care in the more than six hundred homes in B.C. It would also be more costly and more complicated than I could have imagined.

To start, I issued an order compelling all care homes, public or private, to share employee information with the province's Health Employers Association; it in turn would contract a local IT company to compile all the data. This would allow us to understand who worked where and what their wage was. There were over ninety-five contracts for workers in care homes, and we knew already that as many as eight thousand of the thirty thousand workers were employed in multiple places. After gathering the information, we would then sort people based on where they worked the most hours and their preferred care home. Most importantly, the government committed to bringing all workers up to the union wage to ensure that homes were not left wanting. This complex endeavour became known as my "single site" order—and it turned out to be a key measure in preventing COVID-19 from entering care homes in B.C. Not only that, but it would become an important foundation for enhancing the staffing and the prevention of other infections in care homes as well. We were determined to put it in place, not only to ensure that residents of all care homes in B.C. received the care they needed, but that homes could safely start allowing family and other essential visitors to come back. It wasn't only about care; it was also about quality of life for our most vulnerable.

These were the issues swirling around me during my first full week in Victoria since January. Underneath the whirl, I felt a profound sense of relief not to be flying back and forth to Vancouver. Despite the ongoing intensity of the pandemic, it somehow seemed more manageable to be based close to home. And my sister Lynn was still visiting, so I had some comfort in that. My days continued to start early and finish late, but my triangle of activity narrowed to home, my office, and the legislature where we had our press briefings.

SOMETIMES IT WAS THE SMALLEST things that made my days bearable. Most mornings my walk to work was in the dark, cold rain that is so emblematic of the West Coast winter. And most mornings I was also on calls with senior government leaders or WHO teams. Juggling my phone and headphones while walking and carrying my bags was a challenge; on more than one occasion I had to drop bags, calls, or both. So during that first week back in Victoria, on a day when I received a pair of earbud Bluetooth headphones, my life became suddenly, immeasurably better. Such a simple thing, too. Now on my morning walks I was able to look around me and once again be reminded that, despite the global chaos this virus had foisted upon us, I could still take a minute to appreciate the cherry blossoms in bloom, to take a deep breath, to hold family close.

As everyone adjusted to the pandemic measures, I chose to relay those thoughts in our daily briefings. It's still important to hug your family or your close friends, I said. It was important, necessary even, to go outside daily if you could, to move, to greet your neighbours—from a safe distance—to let children run and dogs walk. We needed these acts and moments for our mental as well as our physical health. We also needed to find ways to let art or music or dancing or singing— or drag, if we wished—into our lives in a safe manner. I was constantly amazed at the inventive ways people came up with to find a sense of community in virtual and distanced contexts.

This would be essential to see us through, and to support those who were suffering in ways big and small, visible or hidden.

I also knew that in times of crisis people often turn to faith leaders for solace. During the SARS outbreak, when this had become apparent early on, I'd met with leaders of all the faiths in Toronto to help find ways in which communities could come together and support each other safely. Now I arranged for a meeting of faith leaders across B.C. with Premier Horgan and Minister Dix. Over 150 leaders from around the province, of all faiths—Christian, Jewish, Hindi, Sikh, Buddhist, Muslim, and more—called in to our session. I began by acknowledging the vital role they played in their faith communities during this unprecedented time. Then I provided details on the risk groups for COVID-19 so that they understood why I was asking them to modify services to protect people in their congregations. I asked that they consider ways to virtually support people to connect and receive the faith services that would be so necessary during the coming months—and to make it okay, particularly for the elders and seniors in their faith, to participate remotely. I was aware that many faiths supported their communities in other ways, too—specifically by providing meals for people in large congregate settings. So I asked the leaders to revise how they did this as well, and to use the guidance we'd developed for restaurants and food banks to modify these essential services, moving to single servings and pickup or delivery to families and people in need. The important communal meals would also need to be modified in order to keep people safe.

The premier, the minister, and I fielded many questions and concerns. But we also witnessed the faith leaders' overriding sense of responsibility for and commitment to supporting their communities during this time. In follow-up calls over the coming weeks, again I was amazed at the imaginative ways in which these leaders had connected with their communities when they were needed most. Some even reported that their congregations had expanded exponentially: with services available online now, they were accessible to many more people. For once, a happy and positive unintended consequence of our COVID-19 measures.

BY THE LAST WEEK in March, the minister and I were ready to present our data and modelling to the public. In concert with my team and our dedicated colleagues at the BCCDC, we'd developed a presentation that showed the epidemiologic data, the models we used to plan for the health system, and the models we used to gauge the impact of the virus in B.C.

It was undeniably a risk to present the details as we knew them at that time. Our cases were still climbing; our numbers were worrisome. But I was confident that being open and transparent would build trust, and that people would understand the nuances, or at least a good proportion would. Nuance is always a challenge in a crisis, when people crave black and white; they want to know with certainty what to do and how things will play out. I would try to communicate that we were in a place with shades of grey, that we couldn't know with certainty what would happen, but that we were looking at the odds—and here is what we did know.

The deputy and I started the week by presenting the information to the government so that all the ministers would be informed in advance and able to ask questions. We then presented to the two opposition parties so that they, too, would have the details and a chance to understand and question us. This was in line with a pattern we'd established from the very beginning. After all, this was a crisis with implications above and beyond the political realm, public health itself was non-partisan, and we needed to include all parties in supporting their communities. Our presentations to all the members of the legislature that day, government and opposition alike, was met with keen interest along with some trepidation. The very real representation of the data and the curve was sobering to us all, and the questions that arose from all sides were thoughtful and concerned.

Finally, on the morning of Friday, March 27, before the public presentation that afternoon, we had a ninety-minute technical briefing with the media. That way they could see the material in detail and ask questions off the record to better understand and, I hoped, better report on the findings. Then we walked down to the press theatre in the legislature. It was time to talk to the people.

I was anxious about getting it right. As a longtime data nerd I had confidence in the numbers and familiarity with the analysis, especially with using models, but I wasn't as confident in my ability to present all this in a way people would relate to. The idea was that I would explain most of the data and models while the minister would present the health system planning models. The epidemiology was new and important: these were the numbers we followed and presented every day, but we hadn't yet pulled the aggregated numbers together publicly and explained their meaning.

I began with the geographic spread of the virus—the numbers by health authority, shown on a map. It was a surprise to some that every health authority had cases; presenting the daily numbers could sometimes overshadow the key fact that yes, the virus could travel everywhere. Then I presented the data on who was getting infected: 50 percent men, 50 percent women; average age in the fifties. Digging deeper, more women were affected in the thirty-to-fifty age group, reflecting the preponderance of cases among healthcare workers in long-term care. The average age of people in hospital was much higher—in their sixties—while those needing ICU care were mostly in their seventies, with more men than women in hospital. The age of those who'd died was another decade higher: mostly people eighty years old and above, sadly reflecting that our pandemic was focused in long-term care homes.

Next I put up two epidemiologic curves, and explained that the first was by test date and the second, more significantly, by symptom-onset date—information that helped us determine who was at risk of exposure and where someone might have acquired their infection. These data showed, in stark fashion, the progression of our pandemic in British Columbia in a way most people hadn't seen. Then I presented a visual of where, broadly speaking, people were being infected: most infections were linked to a known case, or cluster, or outbreak, while there was still a good proportion of people who'd acquired their infection from travel.

The minister was up next with the hospital planning models. We'd based their data on hospitalizations, ICU stays, and ventilator needs from Hubei, from Northern Italy, and from a recently published paper citing even more severe stats from a hospital in Italy. Then we'd adapted the numbers to B.C.'s population and demographics. We'd then measured our current hospital capacity—along with plans for augmenting it—and compared this to the scenarios from those places that had seen such a dramatic, overwhelming surge. The bottom line was that, given the measures we'd already taken to decant hospitals and postpone non-urgent surgery, we were confident we could weather a storm equal to those experienced in other places. Again, the numbers were stark. But we reinforced our determination to do everything in our power to avoid the worst-case scenario, and express that if we did experience such a wave, we were prepared for it.

Finally, I presented what's known as "dynamic compartmental models"—ones that looked at our cases, how many contacts they had exposed, the mobility of people in our province, and other inputs to give a sense of where we could be heading. This was our "curve." I explained that the models didn't *predict* where we were going but rather gave us a glimpse of the potential scenarios. The curve showed we were on an upswing, but one that in the past week had been ever so slightly slowing. This was our time and our chance: if we all paused and stayed apart as much as we could, we had the opportunity to bend the curve and prevent the worst-case scenario we were planning for. It was up to us.

The flurry of questions that followed focused on several topics, but the one that stuck with me was the repeated call to estimate the number of deaths we would see. The modelling team and I had thoroughly reviewed different models and had unanimously rejected the standard ones—the ones that projected deaths based on statistics from other places. I knew that death was an event that was dependent on our response: on our ability to prevent transmission—particularly in long-term care—and to prevent the overwhelming of our health system. We would minimize deaths if we could ensure that everyone who needed hospital and ICU care could get it, if healthcare workers were protected, and if we could prevent the virus from entering our care homes. That would be our overriding focus.

This was a position I would stay strong on. Every single death was a tragedy I felt deeply, and I know the minister shared this sentiment. Protecting our seniors and elders, ensuring that they knew their lives were valued as keepers of our history and our culture, was central to our response. We could not in any way claim success if our rate of death was merely lower than what other places had experienced.

It was also a position that put me and my team at odds with most others in Canada, and elsewhere in the world, who would subsequently present models that projected death rates. But I believed it was the path we needed to take, and in this I was firmly supported by the minister and deputy minister.

That evening I arrived home exhausted, but also hopeful. Now that the information was out there, and everyone had the same data and models we had, maybe we could fight this together. Maybe we could hold the line—now that people knew what the line actually looked like. My sister came home to find me lying on the living-room floor, still in my work clothes, too tired to move. She ordered takeout from my favourite restaurant and poured me a glass of wine, and for an hour or two I almost relaxed. But that night, the spectre of the next few weeks, and how critical they would be, whirled ceaselessly through my mind.

THAT FIRST WEEK OF APRIL, as we were all holding our collective breath, the downside of the orders I'd put in place came home in a non-urgent but awkwardly personal, surprisingly affecting way (perhaps because it was a sign of how much all our daily lives had changed)—one that I knew would be familiar to many others in the province, the country, and indeed around the world.

When I'd ordered all hair salons closed, it was right at the time I would have normally gone for my regular appointment. Three weeks later, my hair was a COVID-19 mess, becoming more and more unruly for my daily press briefings. So I sent my hair stylist a note asking for help. She did offer to come over and do a cut outside in my garden, but as tempted as I was, I knew it wouldn't be right. How could I, who had asked so much of the people of B.C., bend the rules for my own personal vanity? Instead, my stylist dropped off some products in my mailbox and sent me a sweet video with instructions.

In retrospect, perhaps I should have just waited it out. (Earlier that week I'd even read an article listing the top ten things not to do in a pandemic; number one was cutting or fixing your own hair.) Instead, with my sister's help I attempted to follow the video, trimming and adding highlights to my hair. The results were a clear reminder of why I was a public health doctor and not in the hair business. No one will notice, I reassured myself—but that bubble soon burst. After the next day's media briefing, Twitter and other social media lit up with comments, many remarking that I'd gone to see my hairdresser in violation of my own orders. I joked with my team about it the day after that, but I knew I needed to say something publicly or I'd lose credibility. So in front of the cameras that day I began the briefing by acknowledging that I had indeed tinkered with my own hair. I apologized to my hairdresser and acknowledged that I knew this was the number one thing not to do in a pandemic. I declared that I would not be doing it again (for the sake of the rules most importantly, but also, as was clearly by the evidence, for the sake of my hair, too) and I also reassured people that I had not, nor would I, break the rules that I had set. They were there for us all.

———

OVER THE WEEK THAT FOLLOWED, each day brought a roller-coaster of new hope and new challenges. On the one hand the numbers were coming down, lab-testing capacity had increased, and we were learning how to detect and jump on long-term care facility outbreaks rapidly. But other problems were popping up, first among them an outbreak in a federal correctional facility located in B.C. This was something we'd foreseen as a possibility, and had been talking to the federal government to try to prevent it. Meanwhile we'd implemented COVID-19 safety plans in all our provincial correctional facilities and were monitoring them daily. We knew that introduction of the virus into these settings could lead to rapid spread and might well be lethal—another lesson I'd learned the hard way during SARS in Toronto.

Once the cases were detected in the federal facility, we had challenges connecting with the staff and medical team, who weren't accustomed to sharing information with provincial public health. It was only through persistence and insistence that we overcame that reluctance and prevailed in getting infection prevention and control measures to the inmates. In the end, over 60 percent of the people in the facility became infected with COVID-19 and one person died.

Then we had workplaces with cases—particularly among essential workers in poultry-processing plants and fruit-packing facilities. Our teams of environmental health officers partnered with WorkSafeBC to inspect and put in place control measures to stop the transmission. These included erecting barriers, minimizing staff, and providing sick leave support, testing, and masks, all of which helped make these workplaces safer.

As each flame sparked a new fire, we responded quickly and put it out.

As Easter approached, I slowly started to exhale. The numbers I pored over daily were truly and consistently dropping. My colleagues in emergency departments and hospitals were also daring to breathe again. The flood of people with pneumonia and respiratory illness was decreasing dramatically, and hospitals were starting to see the "normal" heart attacks and trauma that always kept them busy. Cases smouldered in some settings, but public health was able to manage these flares; most were people who'd been identified as contacts and had already isolated.

All around us—in Washington State and the rest of the U.S., in Ontario and Quebec, and in the U.K., France, Spain, and Brazil—the pandemic raged. Yet in British Columbia we seemed to be holding our line, bending our curve. Although we couldn't for a moment be complacent, our actions and measures did seem to be working. The people of B.C. had heard the call and had done what was needed to protect both the ones they loved and, equally important in the big picture, the ones they didn't know.

I knew we were a long way from this being over. But we'd found a way to manage the pandemic for now, and without overwhelming our hospitals or locking down our communities. Instead we'd worked together, remaining physically distanced but socially connected.

Or, as I said daily now, by taking to heart the need to be kind, be calm, and be safe.

IN LYNN HENRY'S WORDS

O n Friday, April 4—a Friday only too much like the one
before; the Friday following the end of March, when
British Columbia had presented the country's first public
modelling data for the pandemic—I watched on my phone as
Bonnie answered a reporter's question at the legislature with
one word: "No."

This was followed by a cliff dive of silence: eight full seconds.

The question was, in paraphrase: Will you release a projected death count for our province?

A week earlier, on Wednesday, March 25, Bonnie, now stationed full-time at her office in downtown Victoria, had arrived
home in the evening to her usual suite of before- and after-
dinner calls with regional and national colleagues and with the
province's deputy minister of health. Occasionally the round of
calls also included Bonnie's predecessor and mentor, Dr. Perry
Kendall, who'd recently retired after almost twenty years in the
"top doctor" role. I could tell when Bonnie was consulting with
him by the familiarity and warmth in her voice. These chats
had been more frequent recently, after she had asked him to be

part of a newly funded research initiative—one that, through the Michael Smith Foundation in partnership with government, universities, and other institutes, was studying pandemic responses. She was fond of quoting one of Dr. Kendall's guiding principles: "You can make a point or you can make a difference"— a saying often in her mind now, I knew, as she obsessively tracked the virus's as yet unknowable curve, tried to walk in step with the government while maintaining her autonomy and integrity, and balanced concern with encouragement in her public messages. Neither hope nor fear, on the other hand, was part of the message, although they were often byproducts; another of my sister's favourite quotes was "Hope is not a strategy."

"Okay," she breathed at last, easing off the earbuds she used for calls as I entered the kitchen carrying a large brown paper bag. It was around seven p.m., and by earlier agreement I'd fetched a takeout dinner from a favourite bistro nearby. On the way there, waiting to cross an intersection in the centre of the neighbourhood's little village, I'd caught a phrase wafting out of a passing car's window: "But Dr. Bonnie Henry says . . ." intoned a man's voice. At the bistro, as I stood in line outside the open-air takeout window, I leaned forward to read the menu posted on a sandwich board. Big, bold, script-like letters proclaimed, *Dr. Bonnie wants you . . . to support your local restaurants!* On the way home, seeing that the line outside the grocery store had only two waiting souls, I joined the queue and popped inside to pick up some fruit. At the cash, the young woman behind Plexiglas rang in the dozen apples and oranges as I fished out a cloth bag. She shook her head. "No reusable bags allowed," she said. "I can give you a plastic bag, but I can't fill it for you. You have to take everything outside and do it yourself there. Dr. Henry's orders."

As I awkwardly cradled the loose groceries and left the store, I considered the ubiquity and reach of my sister's supposed orders. "Listen, can you do me a big favour?" I said to her back in the kitchen. "Could you please make a pronouncement about bags at your next briefing? There is much plastic bag confusion out there."

But Bonnie was intent on her laptop screen. "Want to see something?" she said, turning it towards me. An array of brightly coloured graphs and charts featured zigzag lines, a range of peaks and valleys, and a jaggedly uneven wall of bars. "Modelling," she said with satisfaction. She looked up. "This is confidential."

"Of course. Where does it come from? What does it say?"

"I've been working on it with my colleagues at the B.C. Centre for Disease Control," she explained, getting up to find plates and cutlery and pour two small glasses of wine, then two more of water. "A number of the provinces do this kind of modelling—Ontario and Quebec, for example—as well as the federal government. It depends on whether a province has a research arm, like the BCCDC here. In any case, we've all been sharing our data with each other in our calls since early on in this pandemic, discussing what it means. Or what we think it means." She sighed. "You have to remember," she said, in the tone of someone patiently stating the obvious, "there is data. And then there is interpretation. And *then* there is meaning."

My sister turned the laptop back towards herself and scrolled until she reached a particular slide. "Recently, understandably, a lot of people—the press, and also the government and politicians—have been asking if we could do a public presentation of this modelling that we discuss privately in our leadership group. So I said yes. I'm going to do it. This Friday.

But in the meantime, over the past week or so, I've been having pretty intense conversations, as maybe you'd imagine, with my colleagues, those amazing scientists and researchers at the Centre. About how to present the data and how to explain what the modelling means. And this document is what we've agreed on for the press conference. First, though, I have to brief cabinet tomorrow morning. That's what I'm prepping for now. And then I do a separate session with each of the opposition parties."

Now Bonnie turned the screen back towards me. "This one is important," she said.

The single slide on display was simpler, starker, less colourful than the other flashier portraits of our possible future. It showed only one blue line traversing a series of dates—days and weeks—in a lazy arc that reminded me of a casually outstretched arm, or a child's drawing of wind or breath.

"The curve," Bonnie said, cryptically. "Or where we think the curve is pointing. Actually, it's still undecided. What it shows is that the next two weeks or thereabouts will definitely tell the tale."

"And this," I said, "is that curve of virus transmission we all famously want to flatten."

Bonnie nodded and closed her laptop so we could eat.

But the afterimage of that half bow seemed to hover in the air even as the perfectly round disc of the sun outside the kitchen window made a big red show of setting; I imagined the curve's uncertain arc taking the place of the more pointed V for virus that my sister had so vividly described being stamped on her forehead almost two weeks before.

It must have been in her mind, too, because after we'd cleaned up our dinner and she had placed her laptop back onto the table and prepared to settle into a final hour or so of work, Bonnie said suddenly, "You know, I really do believe in giving people the information, telling them why, speaking directly to them—not only to get us through this together, which is the only way through, but to minimize trauma. I think we in public positions sometimes underestimate our fellow humans' capacity to understand complex things. But we're in this together, and I believe we have a duty to share the important information, explain what it means and why, and then give people the means to do what's necessary. To support them to do it. Which isn't to say that the effects and the support are the same for everyone. Don't get me wrong"—this in response to my anticipated caveat; my sister could see me raising a finger to make a point—"I know it's not at all the same for everyone. We're in the same storm, but we're not all in the same boat. Or in a boat at all, in some places. We've already seen how this virus is exposing inequities. But at least we can start with sharing what we know."

The next day, Bonnie did indeed meet with cabinet and the opposition parties. And the day after that, on Friday, March 27, with a kind of sober keenness, she explained what lay in the numbers and spikes, the colours and arches of the charts and graphs scientists used to describe what they had traced, and now predicted, of COVID-19's still unsettled path.

Shortly after, Ontario gave notice of its intent to release similar modelling the following week—and I marked the date with a small shiver. After the Easter long weekend I would be returning home to a no doubt greatly changed Toronto, still shrugging off winter; best to be prepared for what awaited me there.

———

THIS WASN'T THE FIRST time B.C. had led the way with a COVID-19 initiative.

Bonnie had told me about another decision, one that turned out to be prescient, a few days before, after her return to Victoria for good. She had been looking over the daily numbers at home in the morning, while I'd been connecting by email, text, phone, and Zoom with colleagues, who were mostly in Ontario, and authors, who were scattered around the country and indeed the globe. I had just finished texting with a writer who spent part of each year in his birth city of Mumbai—and who, when the pandemic was declared, had made the difficult decision to stay with his parents in the family apartment there rather than return to Canada. I was worried about the news of the virus in India, about the colony of tiny connected homes where I knew he lived in the crowded city, and about him, the only child of older parents. And although his texts sparkled with his usual easy wit and good humour, I sensed a darker undertow. "Are you careful? Do you go out at all?" I asked him. "At night," he replied. "Only at night, after it's dark. I go out to a nearby track and take my mask off and just run around the oval for an hour. I don't see a soul. Then I put on my mask and go back to my parents." For some reason, this news filled me with unexpected grief. I imagined my author—who had often regaled me with stories of his voluble, eccentric extended family and colourful childhood friends in India—running solitary laps under a deep purple sky, grey gravel underfoot, illuminated only by stark fluorescent lights on sentry-like poles.

After our exchange ended, I sat there thinking. Perhaps, I considered, the little note of constant sorrow I'd been feeling was related to this disembodied contact. Suddenly, and for the immediate future, what I (like so many others with access to technology) knew of the everyday lives of friends, family, and colleagues, and what they knew of mine, was mostly light refracted through photos or texts, or sound that arrived phantom-like through a phone, or a combination of image and voice lined up on a screen of tiny people-inhabited squares (each, in a startlingly democratic move, given exactly the same allotment of space no matter their status or position). In this way, while sitting alone on a painted wooden bench tucked into the hollow under a cliff overlooking the Strait of Juan de Fuca, I talked to and imagined a close friend in Montreal sitting on his own solitary metal bench in a little urban park outside a hospital, waiting anxiously for his boyfriend receiving urgent treatment there. And after hearing the ping on my phone announcing the arrival of a photo, I pictured my eighty-year-old father, the source of the image, picking his way slowly and carefully (I dearly hoped) down the sandstone steps in his backyard to check whether the patch of lupins near the apple trees needed watering. Yet how many places and lives went unseen, unheard, moment by moment now?

"Bonnie," I said, "how are things going in the long-term care homes? With the outbreaks, I mean."

"Ah." She looked up from her numbers with a slight frown. "Well, that's a complicated question with a complex answer. The outbreaks are sadly still ongoing. But . . ." She allowed herself a little smile. "There is one thing I'm proud of, maybe prouder of this than almost anything. The minister and I have managed to make sure that the essential caregivers and staff in the affected homes are working in those one spots only. Not only that, we've put in place measures to make sure they're paid equitably across the homes, and at the highest level of the pay grade. That was an issue, and one of the many reasons why

people worked in multiple homes. Now the government is taking it on financially, making it work."

"And the homes without outbreaks?" I asked.

"Yep, we're working on that now, too," Bonnie said. "There
are ninety-something different contracts, and all the variations
between employers and unions and so on. But we're going to
get there. We're determined. And I think Ontario has been taking note. They may try something similar, too."

NOW, ON FRIDAY, APRIL 4, a few days after officials in Ontario
had presented their own modelling data for that province, I
watched as Bonnie's lengthy, loaded silence counted down
uncomfortably. Even the usually expressive sign language interpreter stood frozen in his little inset box. Flashes of the press
briefing in Toronto came back to me: public health officers and
researchers sitting behind a long table as slides—with charts
and graphs similar to B.C.'s, if sometimes with markedly different shapes—appeared onscreen. And the one slide that had
made me catch my breath, a slide unlike any I had seen before,
presented by the CEO of the public health agency of Ontario: it
had announced the expectation that between three thousand
and fifteen thousand Ontarians would eventually die from
COVID-19. That, I remembered thinking, is an enormous, dis-
turbingly hazy gulf between one end of a stark line and the other.

Would Bonnie release a similar slide for B.C.? No.

Into the silence slid all that was unsaid: just because someone had made such projections and calculations elsewhere,
she wouldn't be forced into following suit. Her ideas about the
prediction of such numbers were not the same. Each number
implied a name. And under her watch, there were no reasonably expected or acceptable names.

Later that day, to a journalist, Bonnie would explain her thinking more fully: "We [in public health in B.C.] did not predict the number of deaths. Modelling is not [done] to predict. That is not its purpose.

"You can't predict where [the virus] is going to erupt," she continued. "We all have our own pandemic that we're moving through, and even in different parts of B.C., it's quite different. In the Lower Mainland we know that the outbreak has been driven by, unfortunately, this virus getting into long-term care homes and particularly, too, that it got to [them] very early before it was recognized. You can't model that, you can't predict that, and so that's why I don't feel it's particularly useful to use that as part of our modelling. What we do know is what sort of resources we have to give everyone the best chance of surviving this disease and also to ensure we have the health services and healthcare available for everybody else who needs it at the same time as we're dealing with COVID-19. And that's the approach we've taken here in B.C."

That evening, Bonnie and I strolled together in our little bubble to pick up a pizza at a shop across the park. As we took our place in line, a murmur rippled through the half-dozen or so other patrons, waiting in their six-feet-apart spaces. "Thank you, Dr. Henry," the woman ahead of us said quietly, turning her head briefly to nod.

ON SATURDAY, IN ONE of her rare spare moments, Bonnie gave in to a very personal form of despair—if one mirrored, literally, by millions of individuals around the world, facing their reflections each morning. "My hair," she lamented. "I know it's a weakness. I know I'm the person who closed all the salons. But look at this! And I have to be on television all the time. Whether I like it or not, people notice things about me and comment on them."

"Oh, vanity," I joked, thinking, prophetically as it turned out, of the famous scene in *Anne of Green Gables* where a home dye job goes wrong. "Well, what can I do to help?"

"What I really need is my stylist," Bonnie said mournfully, and for a wild split-second almost appeared to entertain the possibility of arranging to see her. Then she shook her head. "Okay, what I think I can do is ask Lindsay to drop off, distantly and safely, in my mailbox, the stuff I need to do my hair myself." She looked at me significantly. "And then you can assist in our home salon here."

This was one of two lighthearted moments during what had become a dark and volatile early April. The other had happened a couple of days earlier, when my sister had raised her head from a message on her phone with an incredulous, shy, delighted expression. "The shoe designer John Fluevog just emailed me," she said slowly. "He wants to do a special edition shoe in my name." By now, Bonnie was daily receiving cards, parcels, boxes, letters, and countless emails, often with beautiful, heartfelt, sometimes priceless tributes and gifts—even jewellery, as people watched her wear her own colourful and extensive collection of necklaces and brooches in her briefings. Bonnie took delight in the notes and admired each gift but was also careful to respect the government's ethical guidelines around accepting anything of monetary value. She had started a collection that, with the creators' permission, would eventually be part of an auction, with the proceeds going to charity.

The Fluevogs occupied a different category—perhaps a different galaxy—of tribute in my sister's shoe-devoted heart. Bonnie had loved, bought, and worn the Canadian designer's distinctive footwear for years, and when the pandemic press briefings had started up, many people had taken notice—including, eventually, the founder himself. Soon enough, a deal was worked out: Fluevog would produce a limited run of the Dr. Bonnie Henry shoes, with her now inescapable phrase *Be Kind, Be Calm, Be Safe* stamped on the soles, and all profits would go to B.C. food banks, Bonnie's charity of choice, knowing how stretched these organizations were as they supported families in need. (When the shoes eventually went on sale online in May, they sold out in minutes and the traffic crashed the shoemaker's website for hours. In the end, close to 200,000 much-needed dollars were raised for the food banks.)

The experiment in hair was less successful. Bonnie's stylist did indeed leave the ingredients for highlights, along with instructions, in the mailbox. And late on a Monday evening, I did attempt to help Bonnie with the touch-up. But as many watchers of the next press briefing declared, the results were distinctly *browner* than my sister's natural, and usually professionally highlighted, blonde. For about a minute, I found the resulting commentary mildly funny. But soon, and for the first time in my experience (although I now guessed this was not new for Bonnie), a darker, unrelenting, eager chord in the conversation could be heard. Had Dr. Henry broken her own rules? Had she gone to a salon? Had she seen a stylist in person?

This was not innocent or idle speculation. Bonnie was emphatically not a politician, and equally emphatically had no desire to be, but she was under similar scrutiny by the people she served. We were both aware that a number of high-profile politicians, internationally and nationally, had recently bent or broken their own pandemic guidelines—followed by swift and scathing condemnation, and sometimes the loss of both credibility and position.

The avidity of the attention being paid to my sister's hair gave me an odd, dizzy, queasy, frightened feeling, as if peering into a vortex that could swallow you whole. I wondered if Bonnie felt this way much of the time. I dearly hoped not.

The next day she quickly put the matter to rest with a joke, apologizing publicly "to my hairdresser" for the botched job (quickly corrected at home, too, with a follow-up remedy in the mailbox from the stylist).

THE PALL OF DARKNESS over early April had to do with the ever-present, still unpredictable curve of our rate of infection—a ghostly dome over our days and acts, a breath inhaled deeply but not released. The darkness also lay in the bumps and ruptures breaking out along the path of that curve, all of which needed rapid smoothing.

In the March 31 briefing, Bonnie had talked remarkably openly—some in the federal government thought alarmingly so, at least initially, as the issue was a delicate one and potentially involved communities across the country—about the province's first outbreak at a migrant workers' camp and the careful, humane measures that had been put in place to contain it. She and the minister praised the community, in B.C.'s Interior, who had rallied around those essential workers, providing support and compassion. Here was calm, safety, and, perhaps most surprisingly, kindness above all.

Then, as this outbreak was being nicely handled, came news of the first case in a federal penitentiary, one located within B.C.'s borders. Providing care involved navigating layers of government authority, and soon 139 people, 60 percent of whom were Indigenous men, became infected. One man died. In the end, the province worked with the federal government to be allowed to set up a mobile medical unit just outside the prison, and at last the cluster was slowly contained.

One weekend afternoon around this time, as Bonnie caught up on her endless, cascading emails, she suddenly pulled back from her computer in distress and dismay. A man in his early forties had unexpectedly died of COVID at home; he had called an emergency hotline earlier in the day but had appeared at that time to be in no imminent danger. That evening, after Bonnie had cycled through her usual conference calls, we downloaded a movie in a rare attempt at mindless distraction, but Bonnie was as inconsolable as I was numbed by the day's news. "I saw maybe a quarter of that," she said before heading wearily to bed.

Yet as the long Easter weekend—and my return to Toronto that Monday—approached, new light, illuminating new things, crept in around the edges of the lengthening days.

I saw it in little hand-lettered or spray-painted signs on my walks through the ever-changing landscape of the park—so much more alive in this moment than the main commercial streets of the city, which now seemed like phantom limbs full of mysterious, remembered pain. In contrast, the sidewalks in the village and the paved paths in the park were filling up, almost overflowing with multicoloured exclamations and declarations drawn in chalk and paint. Houses were decorated with notes hung in windows or tacked to doors, front gardens displayed sayings spelled out in rocks and seashells. It seemed as though the more virtual our conversations became in this locked-down world, the more these messages appeared, written right on the landscape itself, waiting to be read in unpredictable time by passing strangers. Now when I spotted a phrase chalked on the sidewalk or pinned to a light pole, I felt I was a tiny part of a polyphonic, time-expanded, tactile conversation.

Many of the messages and sayings inscribed on sidewalks and signs quoted "Dr. Bonnie," and I began to take an inventory: there were numerous variations on *Be Kind, Be Calm, Be Safe*, but also *Bend It Like Bonnie* and *Fewer Faces, Bigger Spaces*. And always, simply, *Thank you*.

"WHY DON'T YOU COME with me to the legislature tomorrow?" Bonnie said on Good Friday, arriving home from the office in an unusually buoyant mood. She unloaded briefing papers, newspapers, notebooks, and a bag of cards and letters on the bench beside the kitchen table. "I have to shoot this public service announcement that will air in a week or so. And because it's the Easter weekend, there'll only be a skeleton crew. The minister is still across the water in Vancouver. Last chance to see me in front of cameras before you leave on Monday."

"Sure," I agreed. "You look happy."

"Well, I don't know if happy is right. But . . . it looks like, just maybe, after the weekend—although, of course, we'll need to see the numbers on Monday—we may be flattening the curve. For now."

I opened my mouth to exclaim over this, but Bonnie put up her hand and shook her head. "I really don't want to talk about it yet. I don't want to jinx it. But . . . it looks good."

The next day around noon, Bonnie and I walked in sunshine through deserted streets towards the back entrance of the legislature. Just inside the grounds, my sister paused. We were standing, I saw now, at the start of a flagstone path that wound its way through a modest but beautifully tended garden. Bonnie took a deep breath. "Have I told you about this?" she asked. "Whenever I'm feeling nervous, or really, whenever I come to the legislature before a briefing, I try to walk through here first. I love these roses. You can just see the buds starting over there." She pointed, and I saw that the entire garden was made of rose bushes, all different varieties, each in a slightly different state of springtime life.

Inside the legislature, a camera crew was waiting. I watched, assisting with hair and shoes as needed (in keeping with the physical distancing rules, I was the only person who could come within a metre or so of my sister), as Bonnie thanked the people of British Columbia for helping to "flatten our curve."

Then, as the photographer framed her in springtime pink and green against the high marble dome of the foyer that sloped across to the legislature library, she introduced a new slogan, one designed to help stay the course through the summer to come—and one that would, in time, prove more fitting than any of us peering at her image through the camera's convex eye could have known: "It's not forever, but it is for now."

ON MONDAY MORNING my almost empty plane to Toronto eased into the air just as Bonnie was striding towards her office and the numbers, good ones, that would await her that day. As the plane gained altitude I looked out over the light-brushed water and tufts of land rising from the sea. Everything in the scene below seemed to sway in languid, self-perpetuating, ceaseless movement: the waves, the sunlight, the tops of trees, even the tiny human additions infinitesimally criss-crossing the canvas—ferries and tugs and sailboats and barges; floatplanes and helicopters and, more rarely these days, passenger planes.

The evening before, on an Easter Zoom call, one of Bonnie's friends had told us of a story he'd read about a man who had been running a social media fan club in support of Dr. Bonnie Henry. He had been inspired to start the club when he heard she sometimes received (and, as I knew well, read) critical, angry, even threatening notes from people. This man had no connection to Bonnie other than watching her updates daily and being grateful for how she delivered her news. He wanted her to know that she was indeed appreciated, even admired. But he lived, Bonnie's friend told us, on a remote part of an island, and his internet connection was spotty. Still, as his fan club grew he felt a responsibility to the now thousands of members who had joined. So, every day, once a day, he would climb to the highest point on his island, where the reception was clearest, and manage the new messages and posts.

Now, arching over the last reach of the sea before heading for the mountains, I thought of that man, tapping away on his computer at the very top of his little island, making that daily pilgrimage to connect with like-minded others—out of kindness and fellowship and hope, perhaps. Already it seemed to me like a scene that could belong only to the rapidly disappearing world below. I adjusted my mask, closed my eyes, and settled back sleepless in my solitary row, knowing I would land soon enough in evening darkness, into a different storm.

EPILOGUE

"It's Not Forever,
But It Is for Now"

IN LYNN HENRY'S WORDS

" I understand calm. I get safe. What surprises me is kind. Where does 'kind' come from? How did your sister come up with the idea of saying that?"

It was mid-May—although I did not know it, only days before the death of George Floyd and the new phase of the pandemic that would follow—and I was speaking on the phone to journalist Catherine Porter from *The New York Times*. In the month since I'd returned to a grimly locked-down Toronto, Bonnie had continued with her regular briefings in gently curve-flattening British Columbia. But her words travelled freely across borders, and increasingly widely, and now the *Times*, from the centre of the crisis in New York City, was preparing a profile.

I was startled to be asked the question, yet it happened to be one I was thinking about. Recently, especially as I listened to the many public health messages coming from all quarters, I had been mulling over Bonnie's catchphrase, trying to understand why it had resonated and why it persisted.

"I asked Bonnie's predecessor, Dr. Perry Kendall, about it," Catherine continued. "And he laughed and said, 'Yes, that's

Dr. Henry all right; it's just like her to come up with that. It's part of what makes her so effective.' But I still wonder, why that word 'kind,' how did she decide on it? What do you think it means to her?"

I considered where to begin. I did indeed know the origins of Bonnie's decision to use the word in her public messaging. It had all started—unsurprisingly to me in hindsight, knowing Bonnie's identification with, and concern over, the suffering of children and teenagers during the pandemic—with a question posed by a young reporter during a Vancouver town hall for school-aged children in early March. This boy told my sister that he'd witnessed some people mocking others who were wearing masks. Although he didn't say so, it was teasing that, in his community at that particular time, likely had a racial edge. What should he do? he'd asked.

Bonnie had acknowledged how difficult it must be to see and endure such acts. "When people are afraid," she explained in her most reassuring tone, "when they're anxious, they don't know what to do with these emotions. So sometimes they lash out at others who they perceive as different, and they blame these other people. But the best thing to do is the opposite of that. Especially now. What we can do is try not to judge each other. We all need to be kind."

My sister was talking about kindness here in simple psychological terms, but I knew her thinking on the matter was deeper and more complex, entwining as it did a lifetime of reading (Camus's *The Plague* had made a great impression years before and remained a touchstone, although now in the context of many other volumes of contemporary fiction and nonfiction) with lived experience (not only witnessing the tendency towards, and devastating effects of, "othering" during past viral outbreaks, but also, I suspect, experiencing a childhood continually on the move with our military family, never in one place for long, the two of us, a year apart in age, observant outsiders sometimes slipping inside one group or another) and, not least, an excellent instinct for rhetoric (honed by her earlier years as a navy doctor, and often sole female officer on board ship, tasked with rallying others around medical orders).

All this had coalesced in this moment, in the middle of the pandemic, so that when Bonnie uttered the word "kind" she meant something far removed from, for example, the pop-culture talk-show conceit of showering strangers with unexpected largesse or self-promoting "niceness." I also knew that for her, any act of kindness was the opposite of random or whimsical. It wasn't sudden or fleeting but deliberate, consistent over time, a way of seeing and acknowledging the fellow human in front of you. In fact, *being* kind wasn't so much an act as a rather demanding practice.

Bonnie had told me that it was in March, after the exchange at the children's town hall, when she began to think seriously about finding the right words for a simple but effective message, one that might focus people less on fear and blame and more on how restraining our judgment of others, whose lives and pressures we cannot fully understand, would help us through what was to come. But she was convinced the message would not be effective if it was only a flat exhortation to *be* one particular thing or to *do* one particular thing. There had to be a progression of actions: directed outwards to others first, then inwards to one's self, and finally broadening out towards a shared greater good.

In the days leading up to Bonnie's March 17 declaration of a public health emergency, she turned possible phrasing around in her mind. "I thought about calm," she told me, "because people tell me they admire how I sound calm and that it makes them feel calm, too." She added, smiling, "I even liked the idea it was contagious—in the best way. And then I figured out that the final piece should be safety. The idea that there are things we *can* do to be safe—that we have the agency to do them, that it's in our power to decide to do them. But it wasn't until the meeting before the press briefing on that day, the 17th, when I was scribbling my notes on a piece of paper in the minister's office, that I saw how it fit together."

Be kind. Be calm. Be safe.

Back in Toronto, as I thought more about this refrain, I began to see why its combined effect was greater than the sum of its parts: there was the pleasing rhythm of three, the repetition of the aspirational "be," and the crisp consonance of "kind" and "calm." But also, critically, there was indeed a subtle, implied connection between the phrases, and as Bonnie had intended, a logical progression. Without kindness there was no calm; without kindness and calm there could be no safety. The other thing that struck me was that "be calm," far from being a command directed at others, suggested an internal injunction—to be conscious of your own self, to direct your own life and actions. Whereas kindness, in Bonnie's pandemic-times dictionary at least, wasn't meant as a version of self-help but instead allowed space in the world for others and their lives, even if those lives were not immediately known or accessible to you. From this emerged a fragile shared safety in an alarmingly unsafe world.

I said some of this to the reporter, who listened intently, recording it all, and went on to write her article. But between that interview and the publication of the piece in early June, I found myself thinking again about those three words when

George Floyd's breath and life were unconscionably ended on May 25. Of what use was calm now (and who among us should be calm?), or safe (and who among us were the safe ones?), or above all the anodyne-sounding kind?

Around that time, Bonnie sent me a text. "I'm trying to come up with a metaphor we can use publicly for this stage we're in now with the pandemic," she wrote. "But I definitely don't want to use war or military imagery." As I waited for her to type her next message, I nodded to myself. Politicians in the United States were using such comparisons with abandon; the further one's distance from that, the better. Another whoosh on my phone. "What do you think?" the next text read. "Something to do with nature, maybe . . ."

I considered the options. Fire, perhaps? But no: "fighting fire" has a particular meaning in British Columbia, and all along the west coast, where raging wildfires have become an almost yearly trauma. Plus, it didn't feel true to the nature or course of the pandemic as it was unfolding. Likewise, flood wasn't right, nor was hurricane; both were again too specific, too contained in their consequences. We agreed finally that probably the best metaphor—the one Bonnie would go on to discuss with her team—was the more general "storm." A storm could pass through phases over time, it could take on different forms, and it could have a variety of effects on different people and populations and places. Yet it would spare no one entirely. No matter who and where you were, you could imagine yourself in this storm.

As we ended our exchange, I asked my sister if she was still using her most famous catchphrase to end every briefing. "Yes," she texted. "It endures. Just like us."

That was when I remembered, with a jolt of surprise, that Bonnie's idea of "kind" was, in fact, related to the word's socially complex root: "kin." Kin was, frankly, a word I felt ambivalent about, having reflexively associated it with a dangerously restricted circle rather than an open one. But now, imagining it illuminated by "kind," I considered the opposite: that it was an open word, not a closed one; expansive, not limited. That we ourselves could choose its nature and meaning. Especially, necessarily, even urgently, now.

Barbadian prime minister Mia Mottley's clarion call for change echoed back to me now, too, from the time before this time, that vanished moment when my sister and I, "kin" who'd found ourselves unexpectedly in each other's company, were poised between the old year and the new. The night sky I'd thought so soft and quiet back then had really been ringing with voices, calling out into the coming storm. *We must have caring and empathy . . . It is not about governments anymore. It is about people. I ask this global community to pause. Time is running out.*

Finally, I recalled something I had somehow forgotten in the many distractions of the past weeks, something that Bonnie had told me once, over the phone, was the final piece clicking into place as she'd created her refrain—the coda she had created then too, and would wait to use when the moment came and it was most needed.

"I believe we need hope, too," she said. "For me, 'be kind' fosters emotional well-being and gives people a sense of belonging; 'be calm' is about mental well-being and gives meaning; and 'be safe' is about physical well-being and gives us a sense of purpose."

She paused, and I could hear her move to the fridge and pour a glass of something. Then her voice, measured and sure in my ear. "But there's something else. The only thing that will get us through: something that looks further ahead than being kind and calm and safe, further than the emotional, mental, and physical. Something that looks beyond the now, and everything we're required to keep doing in this time. You can call it hope. Or faith. Whatever you name it, it has to do with the spirit. I wanted some words to say, Yes this is hard, and yes it's a long road—but it isn't forever. This time, too, will pass. That's why I came up with a fourth line to add sometimes—for the sake of hope. Be kind, be calm, be safe. And: It's *not* forever . . . but it is for now."

IN DR. BONNIE HENRY'S WORDS

I t is not forever. . .but it is for now.

Fall is now approaching. And as I look back at the last nine months, at COVID-19's tragic, far-reaching effects, in some ways it all seems overwhelming. I am also struck by how much we have yet to learn. Who knew when 2020 dawned that we'd see so much change sweep the world, and so quickly? This storm that has overtaken us has, in its upending of all that was customary in our lives, exposed many things, the primary one being that we're connected, a global community in ways we perhaps hadn't appreciated or perhaps had ignored. We've learned that what happens in an unfamiliar city in China affects us; what happens in Iran affects us; what happens in Washington State and Oregon and California and New York and Florida affects us.

We've learned so much about the virus itself, yet our responses to this knowledge haven't always been even and measured—and this too has been a revelation. We've seen responses defined by geography, poverty, politics, bravado. That the U.S. and U.K., supposedly the most prepared countries on the planet, struggled and still struggle even as Hong Kong and Korea and Singapore weathered the storm; that people in Brazil and India suffered and still suffer immeasurably—much of this took us by surprise. And now, with fall coming and cases again climbing globally, we're entering the unchartered territory of a second wave while still rattled and challenged by the first.

HERE IN BRITISH COLUMBIA, as I look back across that long stretch of days from March to mid-April, I see that we had indeed flattened our curve—and, by virtue of our individual and collective measures, kept it down through the spring and most of the summer.

There were, however, a number of discrete outbreaks along the way, some in long-term care homes, and some in workplaces where it was a challenge to keep people physically distanced; these included several poultry-processing plants whose employees worked shoulder to shoulder in a cold, close environment. We also had a large outbreak in our province's farms among temporary foreign workers, obliged as these expert employees were to live in crowded shared accommodations. COVID-19 revealed the plight of these workers, from Mexico, Guatemala, and Vietnam, who'd been coming to Canada, some for years on end, to provide the essential skilled farm labour we couldn't find at home. Eventually, upon their arrival here they were housed individually in Vancouver hotels for the duration of their incubation period, with access to testing and support should any become ill. And indeed, over the course of the spring and summer over sixty of these workers tested positive while in quarantine, a reflection of the risk now ongoing in their home countries. We made sure they received the care they needed, in the process preventing what could have been many more out-breaks across the province.

From every one of these outbreaks we learned what mea-sures worked to limit employees' exposure and to control viral transmission: physical barriers, physical spacing, small work pods, PPE (especially masks), and reduced contact in shared accommodation. Environmental health officers teamed up with inspectors from the province's workplace safety agency to scruti-nize all other similar premises around B.C. and implement safety measures. As well, we required that large industrial camps, often in remote areas of the province, develop COVID-19 safety plans to protect not only their workers and worksites but also the people nearby, many of them First Nations communities.

We had successes. For example, among the thousands of workers planting trees across the province's north and interior, in places devastated by wildfires, not a single COVID-19 case was found. We kept construction projects going, ensuring that much-needed seniors housing and hospital projects could progress. And among the over ten thousand temporary foreign support farmers around B.C., no further outbreaks occurred.

By the end of May our community transmission was low enough that we were able to reopen schools for the month of June—and although on a limited, voluntary basis, with online instruction continuing, that reopening was important. It was important for lessening the fear that had developed around schools and for trying out protection measures that would work in the fall. It was also important for giving young people a sense of closure, especially those in grade twelve who were leaving their classrooms for the last time. In all, about a third of the province's children, over 300,000, returned for at least some time in June. And although we had two exposures, from attending school during their infectious period, no transmissions ensued, and no outbreaks.

We did not, however, get the summer reprieve I'd so hoped for. COVID-19 risk continued unabated, with cases surging in Washington State and across much of the U.S. Everything COVID-19 had become political there, from mask wearing to testing to treatment. And that meant increased risk for a surge in Canada as well, since, of course, when the virus spread anywhere, the risk was everywhere. My hope that the warmer weather and the waning of influenza might mean this coronavirus would subside also did not prove true. With so many susceptible people, the virus re-emerged whenever we gave it the chance.

Still, in May, we began our cautious, gradual reopening—a measured operation that would allow us to identify and respond to surges quickly and rapidly stop outbreaks. I'd been thinking about this from the moment we had put measures in place in March. Knowing that the restrictions and isolation measures we implemented would have unintended consequences, some perhaps positive but many negative, and that we needed to keep the fewest restrictions possible in place for the shortest amount of time, I'd set up a team to quantify these unintended effects; we used the resulting data to inform our plan to restart our world. After all, a healthy community meant more than just its physical health. There were also urgent economic and social issues that contributed to health: workers losing their jobs, parents struggling to play the role of teacher and entertainer while trying to work from home, single people not having the community and physical connection we so need as humans, families getting cut off from their loved ones in hospital and long-term care. These consequences, along with the uncertainty of how long it all might last, would take its toll on our collective well-being.

The plan was for the restart to be one-way only—to find that balance between maintaining protective measures while resuming our lives: businesses open, surgeries and health services back to full capacity, restaurants and hair salons and retail stores back, but with measures in place to keep people safe. We created a bigger "safe reopening working group" that connected with the different sectors and developed guidance for each type of business to use. I issued an order that every business would need their own COVID-19 safety plan that must be available to both employees and the public.

Slowly and surely we moved into the light. Stores reopened with space requirements, customer limits, and masks. Restaurants reopened with Plexiglas barriers, small numbers, spaced tables, and for many, outdoor patios. Long-term care homes now allowed in a single visitor to see their loved one, complete with masks and distancing; it wasn't perfect and not nearly enough for the many families who'd been separated for so many weeks, but it was a start, and one we believed would be sustainable into the fall and respiratory season.

WE'D ALSO LEARNED, HOWEVER, that although we're all in the same storm, we're certainly not all in the same boat. Inequities that exist in every nation had been laid bare: racialized people, Indigenous people, women, and those with lower incomes suffered more—not only from COVID-19 itself but also from the measures we imposed to quell its spread. While some sailed through with battened hatches, others had been cut adrift or tossed into the seas, clinging to a life ring. The tragic killing of George Floyd affected us here, with Black Lives Matter demonstrations across the country highlighting that this

pandemic was no different from every past pandemic in exposing the underlying systemic racism in many of our institutions,
from police services to healthcare. Indeed, although the term
"unprecedented" has often been used to describe this pandemic, in so many ways it was indeed "precedented." History
has shown that pandemics are not only inevitable but harder
on some groups than on others. And in Canada, influenza,
smallpox, and TB epidemics have been particularly cruel to
Indigenous peoples. As Heiltsuk elder Pauline Waterfall has
cautioned us, to subscribe to this notion of unprecedented is
to deny or negate the previous pandemics and traumas that
First Nations peoples experienced historically. "This is not an
unprecedented time for us First Nations who have gone
through many challenges and changes that have forced us to
be strong, resilient, and adaptive." She reminds us that we
must acknowledge this in our continued response to COVID-19,
and that we must act in the true spirit of reconciliation to over-
come these inequities.

And in this extraordinary, challenging year, young people
too have particularly suffered, facing greater uncertainty—
both in their access to jobs and in their university experience,
with most postsecondary institutions moving to online-only
courses—right at a time in their lives when forging connections with others is such an important part of their growth. So
it was perhaps inevitable that as the summer progressed they
would find ways to be together, which in turn inevitably led to
an upsurge in viral transmission. In B.C. this was most evident
after the July 1st long weekend in the Interior when hundreds
of young people met up at cottages and resorts, leading to a
spike in cases a week later. Reluctantly we put another order in
place to limit visitors to rental places, and for the first time the

Ministry of Public Safety imposed fines for those who broke the orders. A few high-profile fines in the next few weeks seemed to settle things down.

By late August, however, our numbers in B.C. had started to rise and my gnawing anxiety had returned in full. I knew we needed to focus on regaining a balance between controlling the number of cases in the community and ensuring the all-important opening of schools. For, of course, it wasn't only our young adults who'd been hit at a vulnerable stage in their lives; our children, too, were suffering. We heard from families across the province—and in every income strata, neighbourhood, and race and ethnic group—that children were struggling and falling behind in their education. Calls to the kids' helpline had soared; anxiety and mental health concerns had increased dramatically. And we knew all too well that for some children, school represented a safe haven and a place where they had access to food, social services, and even healthcare. We also knew that this was an especially challenging time for children with special needs, as these services were almost all delivered through the schools and there had been no way to provide them in the lengthy time away from the classroom. In short, the safe reopening of schools needed to be a priority. And since this would facilitate parents getting back to work, the health and well-being of everyone depended on finding this delicate balance.

OUR SUMMER HAD BEEN marked by new challenges as public health teams moved to put out each successive flare-up. The virus was in our community; all around us we could see that when our attention wavered it would spread rapidly. Meanwhile, the media repeatedly asked me the question that was on everyone's mind: Would there be a second wave—and would it overwhelm us, force us back into the dark, lonely existence we'd just survived? I couldn't know what would happen, but I did know that every other pandemic in recorded history has had a second, and, in some cases, a third or fourth wave—and that the second wave was often the more severe and deadly. I also knew that influenza season would return in the fall and that respiratory viruses would begin to circulate once the weather started to cool. With COVID-19 now circulating, even at low levels, it would become increasingly hard to tell the difference between it and the other causes of coughs, fevers, and cold symptoms. And we knew for certain that influenza would lead to outbreaks in long-term care and would stress our healthcare system, just as it did every year.

We had to prepare. We needed the testing capacity to distinguish between COVID and influenza; we needed to ready our health system so that we could withstand a surge without having to shut down the province; we needed to ensure sufficient PPE stocks; we needed to recruit and manage those trained in public health to find every case and contact.

I knew it would be that much more difficult this time around. Over the summer people had had a taste of freedom, so having them return to a fastidious observance of pandemic protocols would be challenging. But I also knew that, as we moved increasingly indoors once the rains and cold began, we'd need those safety measures more than ever.

For our dark spring had taught us that individual actions do make a difference. That the things we did to keep ourselves and our loved ones safe were also the very things that kept our communities safe. Every time we maintained a safe distance, wore a mask, cleaned our hands, and stayed home when we were sick made a difference for those we were closest to and for our community, for those we loved and for those we didn't know. People had mostly responded to our calls to bend the curve, not the rules, and to physically distance and socially connect. We in B.C., and in the country as a whole, had weathered the storm so far by doing our bit individually—and therefore, collectively, we benefited.

Over these months we'd also learned that crises such as this pandemic can bring out both the worst in human nature and, fortunately, the best. Throughout history, social responses to disease outbreaks have encompassed both those poles of human response, including, for some, a focus on prevention and anxiety control; for others, avoidance and denial; and for still others, flight and escape. Historically, some turn to blaming, scapegoating, and stigmatizing, and this is something we've seen now and here too, whether the target has been Asian Canadians or those with U.S. licence plates. But pandemics can also lead to altruism, which we've seen in such acts as dropping food off for neighbours, caring for others' children, and supporting the food banks.

I'd learned that tipping people towards such kindnesses was one of the important roles I needed to play. We'd seen that when there are many unknowns, as there were in January, February, and March and even to some extent today, misinformation and fear can easily fill the gaps, fed by our own experiences, rumours, the media, and, of course, social media. And so I'd hoped that, by providing people with all the information they needed and by emphasizing a shared, collective effort rather than enforcement, we could prevent the more extreme responses and foster the best. I believed that by recognizing our need for connection, compassion, and community, acknowledging that we're in this together, and cultivating a sense of common purpose we would build a resilience that would support us all through this storm.

AS WE HEAD INTO the fall, I'll need to rely on that trust and resiliency we've developed, knowing that we're all weary, that pandemic fatigue is very real, and that more than anything we all just want to go back to normal—the old normal, not this new and tiresome one.

I also think of all that we have learned in these months, from new habits for staying safe to the new words and phrases that have taken up a place in our lives—among them epidemi-ological curve, contact tracing, non-medical masks, essential worker (which now includes grocery store clerks, truck drivers, and garbage collectors), PPE, nasopharyngeal swab, bend the curve, lockdown, two metres/six feet, 'social' and then 'physical' distancing, bubble, quarantine, and Zoom (with its inevitable "You are on mute").

We have learned the true value of toilet paper. We've learned that you should never ever do your own hair in a pan-demic. But we have also learned that we can be resilient and adaptable, even when it's hard. That social connections, even when virtual, are essential. That compassion is stronger than cynicism. That even when faced with unrelenting uncertainty, there is still joy and beauty in the world. As Albert Camus wrote in *The Plague*, "what we learn in a time of pestilence" is that "there is more to admire in men than to despise."

COVID-19 may define 2020, but it will not define *us*—we will, assuredly, go on into a different future. This pandemic, and all we must do to weather it, won't last forever—but it is for now. It is our community and compassion that will see us through this storm, and in the meantime our task for our future is becoming ever clearer: in the same way that past pandemics have led to fundamental change, we must find the means to build back stronger and more just.

But for now, as I imagine that future from the middle of this storm, it remains our time to be kind, to be calm, and to be safe.

ACKNOWLEDGMENTS

DR. BONNIE HENRY

This book is the brainchild of my brilliant older sister, Lynn, and I am very grateful for her support, cajoling, and ever-so-gentle pressure to get these thoughts and events down in writing while they were still seared in my memory. These are memories of the events as they unfolded from my personal perspective through those anxious first months of the COVID-19 pandemic; any inaccuracies or inconsistencies are my fault entirely.

I remain very aware that I have unwittingly become the face and the voice of the public health response to this pandemic in British Columbia, and I take this responsibility to heart. I have tried to portray the heroic work of the public health and health care teams in B.C. in that light. I am grateful for, and in awe of, the strength and expertise of my public health colleagues across B.C. and this country; once again, it is our work that will get us through this storm. In particular, I must acknowledge the wisdom and support of first and foremost Dr. Stephen Brown, and also Dr. Perry Kendall, Dr. Danièle Behn-Smith, Dr. Brian Emerson, Dr. Rèka Gustafson, Dr. Alexis Crabtree, Dr. Paul Gully, and my dear friend Dr. Tony Mounts in our many, many conversations in the past months. Thank you as well to Dr. Theresa Tam, Dr. Heather Morrison, and all my CCMOH and PHAC colleagues; this time has been even more difficult than we imagined, and words cannot express my gratitude and respect for all you do. And to each MHO in B.C., and to my brilliant colleagues at the BCCDC, I remain inspired and moved by the exceptional work you do every day to keep the people of B.C. safe; thank you. I am proud and humbled to lead such a formidable team.

Thank you and my eternal gratitude to Laurel Thompson, who I would be lost without, Nicola Lambrechts and Jean-Marc Prevost for your powerful ways with words to support our work and me personally, as well as Amanda, Lucinda, Chris, Hannah, and the entire PHO, MOH, GCPE (health) and HEMBC/EMU team; it has been a most challenging time and you have stepped up in remarkable ways: Happy Day to you all. Finally, to the Honourable Adrian Dix, B.C. Minister of Health, the path has not been easy, but your humanity and compassion (and proclivity for numbers) have been a beacon of light in this storm.

LYNN HENRY

My thanks necessarily start and end with my sister Bonnie. To begin: I thank her for letting me stay like a spy in her home and trail her around, witnessing her work, eventually scribbling notes, and finally pestering her with questions during some of the most sleepless and critical days of her life.

Thanks to our family, especially our parents Susan and William, our sisters Sarah and Jennifer, and our niece and nephews David, Ella, and Fraser, for their support and concern and in some cases, good-natured willingness to make brief cameos in this book. Gratitude to the great writer friends who also make brief appearances: Madeleine Thien and Anosh Irani; and to the great writer friends whose work sustains me daily, and through the years has given me life. To the generous friends and colleagues who offered encouragement and read pieces of the manuscript in progress: John Mackenzie, Shivaun Hearne, Susan Hughson, Laura Repas, Anne Burke, Anne Collins, Louise Dennys, Bettina Schrewe. To Kristin Cochrane for her wise counsel as this project took shape, and to Jackie Kaiser for her deft agenting. To Penguin publisher Nicole Winstanley for taking a chance on a book by a colleague, and to Nick Garrison for navigating the editorial shoals so calmly despite the rapids of our deadline. To our copyeditor Karen Alliston for her laser-sharp eye. To the talented Jen Griffiths for, as always, making the book look good. And thank you to publicist Danielle LeSage, working alongside Nicola Lambrechts on Bonnie's team.

For care of life and limb as I finished this book, I am indebted to the generous folks at the Galiano Inn in B.C., the staff at the Galiano medical clinic, and Dr. Burnett and the surgical team at the Royal Jubilee Hospital in Victoria. Thanks to Pat and Art for aid and kindness and sustenance.

And to end: thank you again to Bonnie, for not complaining when I forced her to spend her first four days of vacation since January writing this book, and still not complaining when my broken arm cut those days short; and most of all for listening when I suggested doing something unexpected at the most inopportune time, and keeping faith we could pull it off together, a pattern established when we were small children and happily continued to this day.